心身医学新理念

袁勇贵　等著

东南大学出版社
SOUTHEAST UNIVERSITY PRESS

·南京·

图书在版编目(CIP)数据

心身医学新理念 / 袁勇贵等著. —— 南京：东南大学出版社，2018.5

ISBN 978-7-5641-7762-1

Ⅰ.①心… Ⅱ.①袁… Ⅲ.①心身医学 Ⅳ.①R395.1

中国版本图书馆 CIP 数据核字(2018)第 087092 号

心身医学新理念

出版发行		东南大学出版社
社　　址		南京市四牌楼 2 号(邮编：210096)
出 版 人		江建中
责任编辑		褚　蔚(Tel：025-83790586)
经　　销		全国各地新华书店
印　　刷		兴化印刷有限责任公司
开　　本		700mm×1000mm　1/16
印　　张		12.25
字　　数		207 千字
版　　次		2018 年 5 月第 1 版
印　　次		2018 年 5 月第 1 次印刷
书　　号		ISBN 978-7-5641-7762-1
定　　价		48.00 元

本社图书若有印装质量问题,请直接与营销部联系,电话：025-83791830

前言

preface

　　近十年来,心身医学在中国得到了长足发展,有数支全国性的队伍在研究和推动着心身医学事业的发展,几乎每周在全国都会有3～4场有关心身医学的学术报告会,心身医学的新理论、新技术也层出不穷。

　　回顾过去的岁月里,我们团队在心身医学相关方面的课题也有十余项,如今将其总结并整理成册,与同仁学习交流,同时也是对我们课题组工作的阶段小结。

　　全书一共分三个部分:新理论、新诊断和新评估。实践是检验一切真理的唯一标准。有些观点虽提出较晚,尚未被权威教科书或诊断标准接纳并获得大家的公认,还需要很长一段时间的反复实践,且还有可能在今后的实践中进一步修正。学术本身是不断发展的,即使修正了,但至少可以让同仁们看到我们理论发展的历程。既然这本书中的新理论来源于临床,就有其存在的道理,我相信临床医生会越来越对这些问题感兴趣。

　　心身医学与精神病学的关系,有人认为精神病学范围大,心身医学是其一个分支;也有人认为心身医学是基础,范围广,而精神医学只是其中的一部分,主要研究精神疾病。其实这两种认识都正确。二者互为基础,只是认识的角度不同罢了。当然,综合医院的心身医学科诊治对象和诊疗模式均不同于精神科,它拥有独特的诊治疾病群:心身相关障碍;独特的服务对象:心身相关障碍患者;独特的诊疗手段:心身诊疗技术(药物治疗、心理治疗、物理治疗);独特的诊疗模式:心身整合整体诊疗模式。因此,心身医学已具备新学科成立的必要条件,成为独立的学科,落到实处,而不只是存在理念中。中国的心身医学科当然要有中国特色,她一定会为实现和满足人民群众日益增长的健康需求而发挥重要作用,她需要得到全社会更多的关注。

袁勇贵

2018 年 3 月 27 日

目录

contents

新评估

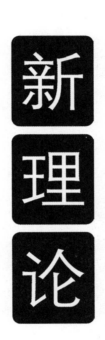

新理论

心身相关障碍的分类与处置

摘要：从心身医学的发展史来看，与"心身疾病"相关的诊断与治疗早已在临床中有所应用。综合国内外相关研究的进展，我们首次提出了心身相关障碍的分类体系，心身相关障碍可分为 5 类，即心身症状、心身症状障碍、心理因素相关生理障碍、心身疾病、躯体疾病伴发心身症状。根据心身相关障碍的疾病特征，提倡对于这类病人实行心身整合治疗。药物治疗、物理治疗和心理治疗"三驾马车"相得益彰地灵活运用，有助于提高病人的治疗效果。

关键词：心身医学；心身相关障碍；心身整合治疗

一、心身相关障碍的分类历史

从心身医学的发展史来看，与"心身疾病"相关的诊断与治疗早已在临床中有所应用。早在 1952 年公布的美国精神障碍诊断与统计手册（Diagnostic and Statistical Manual of Mental Disorders，DSM）第 1 版（DSM-Ⅰ）中即有"心身疾病"这一诊断条目；在 1968 年的 DSM-Ⅱ 中被更名为"心理生理性植物神经与内脏反应"，定义为"由情绪因素引起的单一器官系统的躯体症状"，分类则按累及器官，如哮喘为"心理生理性呼吸系统反应"；在 1980 年的 DSM-Ⅲ 及 1987 年的 DSM-Ⅲ-R 中改为"影响身体状况的心理因素"；在 1994 年的 DSM-Ⅳ 中进一步更改为"影响医学情况的心理因素（PFAMC）"；而在 2013 年的 DSM-5 将其归于"躯体症状及相关障碍"中的"影响其他躯体疾病的心理因素"（F54）中[1,2]。国际疾病分类（International Classification of Diseases，ICD）也曾有"心理生理障碍"及"精神因素引起生理障碍"的分类；ICD-10 不使用"心身的"，不主张多用"心因性"，而将传统的

"心身疾病"纳入"应激相关及躯体形式障碍"[2,3]。

　　我国 1958 年曾将精神疾病分为 14 类,无心身疾病,而 1982 年《中华医学会精神病分类—1981》,首次将"心身疾病"作为最后一类精神性疾病纳入诊断;1989 年的中国精神障碍分类与诊断标准第 2 版(CCMD-2)10 类精神性疾病中,第 6 类为"心理生理障碍、神经症及心因性精神障碍",应包括心身障碍在内,在第 1 类"内脏疾病伴发的精神障碍"中也有一些属于心身障碍的范畴;其后的 CCMD-3 中第 6 类"心理因素相关的生理障碍"包含心身障碍,第 1 类"器质性精神障碍"中也有部分[2,4]。

二、我国心身相关障碍的分类思考

　　综合国内外的相关研究进展,我们考虑将心身相关障碍分为五类(见图 1),包括:① 心身反应;② 心身症状障碍;③ 心理因素相关生理障碍(其中包括:进食障碍、睡眠障碍、性功能障碍);④ 心身疾病;⑤ 躯体疾病伴发心身症状。其中心身反应原则上还不能称为一个疾病,只是一种"反应",是指暂时的生理反应,把那些病程较短(<1 周)的患者归为此类别。

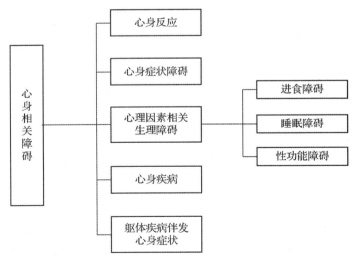

图 1　中国心身相关障碍分类

由图2不难看出,躯体疾病到精神障碍是一个连续的疾病图谱,由躯体疾病向精神障碍的过渡可归纳为包括"心身疾病,心身症状障碍,心理因素相关生理障碍,躯体疾病伴发心身症状"的心身相关障碍移行图谱和包括"躯体疾病伴发精神障碍,应激相关障碍、神经症等,人格障碍、冲动控制障碍,心境障碍,精神分裂症"在内的精神障碍移行图谱。

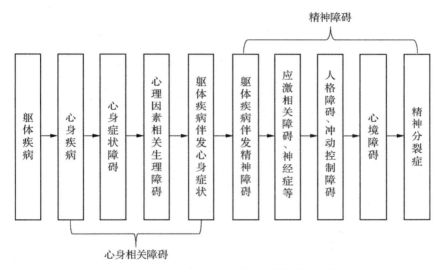

图2 躯体疾病、心身相关障碍和精神障碍的关系

三、心身症状障碍

1. 心身症状障碍的定义

心身症状障碍是一组与急慢性心理社会因素密切相关的综合征,病人具有一定的人格基础,主要表现为焦虑、抑郁、失眠、疼痛、躯体化症状等症状中的一种或几种症状。症状没有可证实的器质性病变作基础,或虽存在一定的躯体疾病,但疾病的严重程度与病人的症状严重程度不相称,病人感到痛苦和无能为力,自知力不全。不符合现有的精神障碍的诊断标准。

2. 心身症状障碍的诊断标准

心身症状障碍需符合下列4个标准:

症状标准(至少有下列一项):① 抑郁;② 焦虑;③ 失眠;④ 疼痛;⑤ 其他躯体化症状等。

严重标准:社会功能部分受损或自感痛苦,促使其主动求医。

病程标准:1 周以上。

排除标准:排除现有的各类精神障碍。

3. 心身症状障碍严重度的评定

见表1。

表 1　心身症状障碍严重度评定量表

条目	评分
应激	0无;1轻度;2中度;3重度
严重度	0无影响;1轻度影响日常生活和工作;2中度影响日常生活和工作;3不能正常生活和工作
病程	0一周以内;1一个月内;2三个月内;3三个月以上

临床医生可根据表1的评定结果,给出具体的建议:轻度(0~3分):可以自我调节;中度(4~6分):建议心身科门诊就诊;重度(7~9分):建议心身科住院治疗或精神科治疗。

四、心身疾病

心身疾病是指具有器质性损害的一类心身相关障碍,往往是指原发性的心身疾病,即心理因素引起的躯体疾病;而继发性心身疾病则是指躯体疾病引起的心理障碍,又称身心疾病,即躯体疾病伴发心身症状。原发性心身疾病,在八大学科中,包括 68 种疾病,具体见表2。

五、躯体疾病伴发心身症状

这类患者的心身症状与躯体疾病紧密相关,它的发生发展和严重程度均与躯体疾病相平行。药物引起的心身副反应也包括在此类中,是指心身症状的出现与消失均与药物的使用密切相关。

表2　心身疾病分类

一、内科	18. 功能性消化不良	36. 帕金森综合征	2. 咽异感症
（一）呼吸系统	19. 肠易激综合征	二、外科	3. 口吃
1. 支气管哮喘	（四）内分泌系统	1. 肿瘤（乳腺癌等）	4. 癔症性耳聋、失明
2. 过度换气综合征	20. Grave's 病	2. 器官移植后综合征	六、口腔科
3. 神经性咳嗽	21. 甲状腺功能减退症	3. 男性不育	1. 牙齿敏感症
4. 慢性阻塞性肺疾病	22. 原发性甲状旁腺功能亢进症	4. 男性性功能障碍	2. 复发性口疮
（二）心血管系统	23. 糖尿病	三、妇产科	3. 扁平苔藓
5. 冠心病	24. 肥胖症	1. 流产	4. 下颌关节紊乱综合征
6. 原发性高血压	（五）风湿免疫系统	2. 异位妊娠	5. 磨牙症
7. 白大褂综合征	25. 类风湿性关节炎	3. 妊娠剧吐	七、眼科
8. 二尖瓣脱垂征	26. 系统性红斑狼疮	4. 胎儿生长受限	1. 原发性青光眼
9. β受体高敏征	27. 雷诺病	5. 胎盘早剥	2. 伪盲
10. 高血压病	28. 纤维肌痛综合征	6. 功能失调性子宫出血	八、皮肤病学科
11. 充血性心力衰竭	29. 白塞氏病	7. 原发性痛经	1. 皮肤瘙痒症
12. 功能性心律失常	30. 干燥综合征	8. 绝经综合征	2. 神经性皮炎
13. 心因性心律失常	（六）神经系统	9. 女性性功能障碍	3. 银屑病
（三）消化系统	31. 紧张性头痛	10. 不孕	4. 白癜风
14. 消化性溃疡	32. 肌痉挛症	四、儿科	5. 斑秃
15. 慢性胃炎	33. （血管性）偏头痛	小儿遗尿症	6. 荨麻疹
16. 溃疡性结肠炎	34. 脑卒中后抑郁	五、耳鼻喉头颈外科	
17. Crohn 病	35. 癫痫	1. 精神心理性耳鸣	

六、心身相关障碍的处置原则

根据心身相关障碍的疾病特征,对这类患者提倡心身整合治疗。药物治疗、物理治疗和心理治疗"三驾马车"相得益彰地灵活运用,有助于提高患者的治疗效果[5]。心身相关障碍的药物治疗临床不外乎四大类,即抗抑郁药、抗焦虑药、心境稳定剂和抗精神病药,如何艺术性地灵活运用这些药物是提高疗效的关键。另外,这类患者往往具有一定的人格特质,药物依从性差,说服其规律用药也与疗效密切相关。当然,中成药对这类患者也有一定的疗效,在临床上患者往往也更愿意接受,临床医生可以合理选用。

既要关注患者的躯体治疗(药物治疗),也要关注患者的物理治疗和心理治疗。物理治疗包括经颅磁刺激、直流电刺激治疗,心理治疗包括认知行为治疗、平衡心理治疗和生物反馈治疗等,关键在于临床医生的合理选用。针对此方面内容的培训也势在必行,这也将是心身医学科发展的重要内容。

参考文献

[1] 美国精神医学学会;张道龙,等,译.精神障碍诊断与统计手册[M].北京:北京大学出版社,2015.

[2] 中华医学会精神病学分会.中国精神障碍分类与诊断标准[M].济南:山东科学技术出版社,2001

[3] 吴爱勤.心身疾病新的评估策略:心身医学研究诊断标准[J].医学与哲学,2012,33(1B):8-10,13

[4] 吴爱勤.心身医学分类诊断评估策略[J].实用医院临床杂志,2015,12(6):1-6

[5] 袁勇贵,刘晓云,陈素珍,等.临床上的疑难杂症与心身疾病[J].实用老年医学,2016,30(9):708-711.

[作者及发表刊物:

刘晓云,胡嘉滢,吴爱勤,袁勇贵.心身相关障碍的分类与处置[J].实用老年医学,2007,31(10):9-11.(有改动)]

中国心身医学科学科建设的思考

摘要： 随着社会经济和医疗卫生事业的不断发展，心身医学逐渐走入人们的视线并越来越得到重视。然而，我国尚未设立独立的心身医学科，缺乏配套的医务人员、治疗模式、组织机构等各方面资源，与当下心身相关障碍大量存在的现状严重不相适应，与国外成熟模式的差距十分明显。本文从心身医学的国际国内现状入手，分析在我国设立心身医学科的必要性，探讨关于建立心身医学科所需要的各方面问题，从而找到中国心身医学科建设发展的方向和路径。

关键词： 心身医学科；精神科；学科建立

21 世纪以来，疾病谱由过去的传染病、寄生虫病和营养不良，转化为以心理社会因素为主要原因引起的心身相关障碍，即心理生理因素共同作用所导致的疾病。据统计，我国综合医院门诊中心身相关障碍占 26%～36%，住院患者的心身相关障碍占了该人群的 79.99%，范围则逐渐扩大到内分泌科、消化科、心血管科、肿瘤科、神经科等临床各科[1]。与心身相关障碍大量存在并严重影响人们健康的现状相反的是，卫计委《医疗机构诊疗科目名录》中并没有心身医学科；全国大多数医疗机构，特别是综合医院并未设立专门的心身医学科室；个别设有心身医学科室的医院，该科室所承担的工作也并非单纯的心身相关障碍的诊疗，往往与心理科、精神科的诊疗领域相混淆。因此，探索我国心身医学科建设的方向，找到其科学发展的路径，对于澄清心身医学与相关学科的界限，增强诊疗心身相关障碍的专业性和有效性，应对当前广泛存在的心身相关障碍问题有着十分重要的理论和实践意义，是当今心身医学工作者刻不容缓的一项工作。

一、心身医学科在国内外的发展现状

（一）心身医学在中国的现状

当前中国心身医学诊疗和研究工作的主要承担者既包括了精神卫生专科医生，也包含具有心身医学知识的临床各科医生。党和政府为了保证人民群众心身健康，也提供了一系列政策支持：2009 年中国卫生部建议三级综合性医院要设立精神科；2012 年 5 月 1 日颁布实施的《中华人民共和国精神卫生法》明确要求综合性医院设立精神科或心理咨询科，处理心身相关障碍、躯体疾病伴发的精神问题；2016 年 12 月，国家卫生计生委、中宣部等 22 个部门印发《关于加强心理健康服务的指导意见》，指出：建立健全心理健康服务体系，加强医疗机构心理健康服务能力，综合性医院要建立多学科心理和躯体疾病联络会诊制度，与高等院校和社会心理服务机构建立协作机制，实现双向转诊。

尽管中医学的思想与现代心身医学有很多异曲同工之处，如天人一体观、形神一体观、整体观等，学术界也有"心身医学起源于《黄帝内经》和《伤寒杂病论》"的说法[3]，但通常认为，现代心身医学于 1984 年才传入中国。我国心身医学科建设在世界范围内起步较晚，无论是团队、主题、研究、法律、组织等各个方面，都与美国、日本等国家存在明显差距。正是由于这些差距，我国心身医学总体上缺乏系统性和专业性，还未形成科学的、固定的模式。

（二）心身医学科的国际主流模式

自 1818 年德国的 Heinroth 最先创造 Psychosomatic 一词开始，心身医学在全世界范围内逐步发展，其概念现已得到普遍认可。心身医学首先从德国诞生，在奥地利得到发展，不久传入美国，然后在日本生根发芽。当前心身医学科的主流模式包括：

德国模式：20 世纪 70 年代的德国，心理治疗特别是精神分析普遍为内科医师所接受，而精神科医师根本不承认心身医学的概念，致使一批以心理治疗为主的内科医师另起炉灶，设立了主要针对进食障碍、神经症性障碍的

"心身医学"，获得了政府对新医学专科的认可。发展至今，在德国的综合医院中，精神科往往与心身医学科并存，服务对象互有交叉，取决于患者是愿意服药还是接受心理治疗。

美国模式：美国很早就在精神科专科医师培训中引入了会诊联络精神病学的内容，并逐渐成为强制性培训核心课程之一。2003年，美国精神科与神经科专科医师委员会正式将"心身医学"作为亚专业，而修完会诊联络精神科培训课程成为心身医学亚专业的附加条件[2]。

日本模式：综合医院精神科医生最早与内科医生合作并成为心身医学会的第一批成员；心身内科学会主要由内科医师和临床心理学家组成；80%的精神科医生更愿意声称自己是"心身内科"医师，这也符合日本医师法的相关规定。

二、设立心身医学科的必要性

虽然我国卫计委医疗机构诊疗科目名录中没有明确提到心身医学科，但其位置基本处于精神科目录下"临床心理专业"的范畴，但这一分类的不科学性显而易见。长远地看，将心身医学科作为一门新学科单独设立，是发展心身医学中国模式的重要途径。

（一）心身医学科不是精神科亚专业

从理论层面看，心身医学是研究精神和躯体相互关系的医学学科分支，是医学的基础，而不是精神病学的分支[4]。实践层面看，将心身医学科作为精神科亚专业对待，既可能引发内科医师对心身医学的忽视，也可能让当前正从事心身相关障碍诊疗的综合科医生无法适应。

（二）目前已具备成立心身医学科的必要条件

心身医学科应当作为临床医学下的独立二级学科专门设立的另一个理由，是其已经具备了新学科的必要构成要素，即具有独特的疾病群体（心身相关障碍）、独特的服务对象（心身相关障碍患者）、独特的诊疗手段（心身诊疗技术，包括心身心理治疗、物理治疗等）和独特的诊疗模式（心身整合整体诊疗模式）。这些独特性将心身医学科与其他学科，特别是精神科做出了显著的区分。

三、如何建立心身医学科

名义上，一个新学科的建立需要相关政策法规的支持，具体说来就是要在《医疗机构诊疗科目名录》中有明确的位置。实践中，医疗机构实际设置的临床专业科室名称不受《医疗机构诊疗科目名录》限制，可使用习惯名称和跨学科科室名称，如"围产医学科"、"五官科"等。在争取政策法规支持的同时，心身医学工作者更应当着重探索并明确其诊疗范围、人员构成、治疗模式、安全管理等一系列建设发展中必须面对的问题，不断健全完善心身医学建设的方方面面。

（一）心身医学科的诊疗范围

一个成熟科室必须有明确的诊疗范围，心身医学科与综合科、精神科既有交叉，又有不同，仅凭综合科医师或精神科医师，都无法完全涵盖心身医学科的诊疗范围。心身医学科诊疗范围如图所示：

心身医学科诊疗范围

综合科医师诊疗范围：
1. 心身反应
2. 心身症状障碍
3. 心身疾病
4. 躯体疾病伴发心身症状

精神科诊疗范围：
5. 心理因素相关生理障碍（进食障碍、睡眠障碍、性功能障碍）
6. 精神活性物质所致精神障碍（烟草、酒精、镇静药物等）
7. 心境障碍（抑郁障碍、双相Ⅱ型）
8. 癔症、应激相关障碍、焦虑障碍、强迫相关障碍、躯体症状相关障碍
9. 性心理障碍
10. 躯体疾病伴发精神障碍
11. 精神活性物质所致精神障碍（如海洛因成瘾等）
12. 冲动控制障碍、人格障碍
13. 心境障碍（双相Ⅰ型）
14. 精神分裂症

图 1　心身医学科诊疗范围

需要注意的是,虽然当前在国内,心身反应、心身症状障碍、心身疾病、躯体疾病伴发心身症状等诊疗对象(图1中1、2、3、4项)名义上被归在精神科诊疗范围之内,但临床实践中,传统意义上的精神科一般不接受这四类患者,精神科的治疗手段对其也往往起不到较好的治疗效果,故上图中未将其列入精神科诊疗范围。

(二)心身医学科的人员构成

科室的人员构成是确保临床治疗效果的重要前提。心身医学科不适合作为精神科亚专业的一个重要原因,就是仅凭精神科医生和护士不能满足心身医学科工作的全部需要。心身医学科不仅需要专业的心身科医生和护士,还需要心理治疗师、心身康复师等配套力量。其中,扮演最重要角色的是心身科医生。根据国际主流模式和我国现状,以及从事心身医学工作所需要的专业知识和技能考虑,学科起步阶段的心身医生的主要来源应当是侧重心身医学研究、接受过心身医学培训的精神科医生。这些精神科医生应当在原有专业技能的基础上,具备更全面的综合性知识,特别是心理治疗、物理治疗、人文关怀方面的知识和技能。

(三)心身医学科治疗模式

随着现代医学已由传统的生物医学模式向社会-心理-生物医学模式转变,心身医学的内涵大大拓展,治疗手段也更加丰富多样,简而言之,应当采用心身整合治疗模式,而非单一的药物治疗或心理治疗。

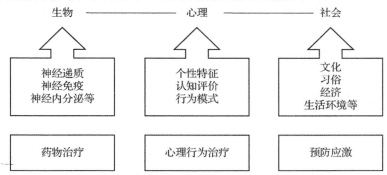

图2 心理-社会-生物医学模式对应的不同治疗方案

图 2 旨在说明，心身相关障碍有综合病因，因此需要综合治疗。心身整合治疗模式的构成实际包含了药物治疗、心理治疗、物理治疗、工娱治疗、体育锻炼等等一系列治疗手段。

对于入院治疗的患者所处的不同阶段，心身科医生也应当开展不同的工作，关注不同的问题，不断完善治疗方案。图 3 展示了心身相关障碍患者在心身医学科住院治疗的阶段模式。

初始阶段	治疗阶段	转归阶段
心理-社会-生物 遗传、生活事件等评估	整合治疗方案	融入正常生活中 开始准备回归社会
明确治疗目标 制订治疗计划 激发治疗动机 健康教育	改变对症状的理解 有效利用各种资源 减轻症状 认识疾病性质	探讨预防复发的方法 开始同门诊医师接触， 计划今后的治疗
同其他患者接触	实践新的应对和 解决问题的策略	治疗结束程序： 走向社会、 回归社会、 服务社会
逐渐习惯各类治疗 以及熟悉治疗师	将家庭成员或 伴侣纳入治疗中	

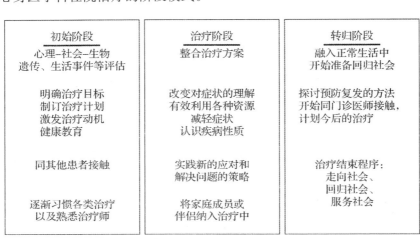

图 3　心身医学科住院治疗的三个阶段

心身医学科病房的安全管理模式应当是内紧外松的。一方面，对医务人员采取内紧式管理，始终把患者安全放在第一位，重视风险评估。严格掌握适应证，不收精神分裂症、躁狂发作等严重精神障碍患者，拒绝收治非适应证患者和高风险患者，如有自杀、伤人倾向的患者。做好全程监控、知情同意、家属陪护等各方面安全辅助措施，确保患者和医护人员安全。另一方面，对患者采取外松式管理，把患者舒适放在第一位，重视心理评估。区分心身科病房与精神科病房的不同，采用开放式病房，以确保去“监狱化”，减少患者的病耻感。

开放式病房对安全管理提出了更高的要求，因此对患者的风险评估不能仅靠医务人员的主观判断，而要通过风险评估工具（如表 1），作出持续反复的科学评估。对于非适应证和高风险患者患者,要及时转诊治疗。

表1　心身医学科风险评估工具

评估项目	分值(0分)	分值(1分)	分值(2分)
入院方式	自愿	部分自愿	不愿住院
情绪状况	正常	兴奋、易激惹或低落	情绪不稳定,有自杀企图
心身症状	症状轻	症状较重	症状严重
合作程度	合作	部分合作	不合作
攻击方式	无	言语	行为
酒、药依赖	无	戒断症状较轻	戒断症状较重
近期负性生活事件	无	影响轻微	严重影响
躯体情况	无	合并较轻躯体疾病	合并严重躯体疾病

(四)心身医学科专科医生培养的课程和亚专业设置

一门独立学科必须有与之相适应的课程设置。"心身医学"提倡健康领域的整体观念和系统思想,关注大脑、心理和躯体的相互作用,研究心理活动与生理功能之间的"心身关系",成为超越精神病学与综合医院各临床学科的医学思想体系[5]。这就要求其课程设置必须涵盖全面,包括:基础课程——普通心理学、社会心理学、发展心理学、心理测量学、心理治疗学;专业基础课程——内、外、妇、儿、口腔、耳鼻喉科、精神病学等;以及最具代表性的专业课程——心身医学。

在此基础上,可以设想,随着心身医学科不断发展完善,将需要在其下设置更为具体的亚专业,比如:综合心身医学专业、心身心脏科亚专业、心身消化科亚专业、心身妇产科亚专业、心身儿科亚专业、心身肿瘤科亚专业等等。心身医学科亚专业设置,既可以在临床上帮助患者得到更为科学合理的治疗,也能在科研上进行更具体的研究,从而达到新的高度。

(五) 心身医学科医生的执业范围和继续教育

在目前情况下,综合心身医学科医生应该具有心身医学和精神卫生两专业的执业范围,可以对精神障碍下诊断;而其他综合科医生,可以在原有的执业范围上,经心身医学培训后增加"心身医学"执业范围,此后,取得"心身医学"执业范围的综合科医生每年要接受一定时数的心身医学和精神病学的继续教育课程,以更新自己的知识结构。例如综合心身医学科医生执业范围包括心身医学和精神卫生;心脏科心身医学专业医生执业范围包括内科(心脏科)和心身医学;风湿免疫科心身医学专业医生执业范围包括内科(风湿免疫科)和心身医学。

四、发展与展望

心身医学在我国尚处起步阶段,其科研领域空白还很多,纵然一些国外的"他山之石"在其本国的研究取得了一定成绩,但是否能够适应我国国情还有待商榷。当务之急需要做好以下几件事:

(1) 获取我国心身相关障碍的基本数据,进行相关研究,如中国心身相关障碍的流行病学调查、中国心身相关障碍的筛查工具的研制、中国心身相关障碍的分类体系及诊疗规范制定、中国心身相关障碍的疾病负担研究等。

(2) 积极创办专门的期刊杂志,如《中华心身医学杂志》、《中华心身医学(电子)杂志》、《中国心身医学杂志》、《Chinese Journal of Psychosomatic Medicine》等。组织编撰《中国心身相关障碍诊疗指南》、《中国心身相关障碍临床诊疗技能培训教程》、《临床心身医学》等工具书。

(3) 在医学院校增设"心身医学"相关课程,在综合科医生的继续教育中增加"心身医学"相关继教课程,提议国家的进一步重视和研究拨款,寻求自然科学基金委员会的研究重点倾斜等,都是我们当前可以做、必须做、要快做的工作。

(4) 培养合格的心身医学科医生、心理治疗师、心身康复师、护士等医务人员,建立成熟的心身医学诊疗模式。

千里之行,始于足下,心身医学科的建设发展任重道远。经过我们的不懈努力,在卫计委诊疗目录中增设"心身医学科"就不是一句空话,定会成为现实。心身医学工作者们要迈开步伐,勇于开拓,努力促成心身医学科的创立,不断推动心身医学在我国的发展,尽快缩小与国际上的差距,甚至赶超国际心身医学发展水平,为心身相关障碍患者谋福祉,为国家心身医学事业的发展做出应有的贡献。

参考文献

[1]　李光英,马东辉,王建.《中医心身医学》教材刍议[J].中国中医药现代远程教育,2013,11(13):100-101.

[2]　于欣.心身医学:从概念到实践[J].中国心理卫生杂志,2009,23(7):470.

[3]　赵志付,柳红良,原晨,等.心身医学理念与中医学一致性的探讨[J].环球中医药,2014,7(10):766-768.

[4]　吴爱勤.心身疾病新的评估策略:心身医学研究诊断标准[J].医学与哲学,2012,33(1B):8-10,13.

[5]　James L. Levenson.心身医学[M].吕秋云,译.北京:北京大学医学出版社,2010.

[作者:袁勇贵　汪天宇　吴爱勤]

临床上的疑难杂症与心身疾病

摘要：临床上疑难杂症并不罕见，且与心身疾病关系密切，约 1/3 的所谓疑难杂症病人可能就是心身疾病患者。目前，综合医院普通科室医生对心身医学和心身疾病的认识和了解仍存在显著不足，且大多数患者又拒绝因躯体症状就诊于心理科或精神科，因此对于此类患者的识别难度较大。作为一个临床医生，应认识和掌握一定的心身医学知识，对于这类患者采取"心身同治"的整合治疗原则以及重视预防此类疾病的发生，从而减少临床上的疑难杂症。

关键词：疑难杂症；心身疾病；心身同治

一个疾病是否疑难，我们能否及时、准确地作出诊断，取决于我们对这种疾病的认识。在临床上，疑难杂症病人常以躯体不适的症状就诊，但是经过针对这些症状进行详细的体格检查或辅助检查，其结果却无异常或异常微小，并且无法解释症状或不足以解释症状的严重程度。

这些机制不明、诊断不清、治疗无效的疑难杂症往往给患者造成极大的困扰，其生活质量也受到严重影响。事实上，这些所谓的疑难杂症患者中，有 1/3 可能就是心身疾病的患者[1]。由于病人不认识、家属不认识、临床各专科医生也不认识，导致病人长期不能得到有效治疗。由此可见，认识心身疾病非常重要。

一、疑难杂症的常见表现

(一) 疑难杂症的危害

疑难杂症在临床工作中并不罕见。Fava[2] 在 1992 年就曾指出综合医院就医人群的 30％～40％具有医学不能解释的躯体症状。在我国，普通人群和在基层医疗机构就诊的患者中，也至少有1/3的患者的躯体症状在医学上无法解释；而且在基层医疗机构中被诊断为精神障碍的病人，有 50％～70％起初都表现为躯体症状[3]。此类患者往往会占用较多的医疗资源，不断奔波于各大医院的各个科室，做大量昂贵的检查、治疗，浪费了大量医疗资源，同时也给自身带来较重的经济负担。而此种情况往往又导致医患双方对诊疗活动均不满意，甚至引起医患矛盾增多、关系紧张。

（二）疑难杂症的常见表现

疑难杂症的症状涉及心血管、消化、神经等众多系统，在众多症状中常见的有胸痛、疲乏、头晕、头痛、失眠、麻木、呼吸困难、腹痛、水肿、体重下降等。病人在描述症状时，表现出焦虑、抑郁的症状，往往会运用"恶梦、可怕"等富含感情色彩的词汇来强调症状严重，诉说这些无法解释的症状严重地影响其日常生活及社会行为。一般来说，这些症状往往是非特异性、模糊多变的，很难具体化，且缺乏肯定的病理生理基础。

（三）诊断和分类标签化

虽然在各科门诊中，以躯体症状为主诉但缺乏客观生理原因的患者相当多见，但在相关的诊断分类上却存在混乱与不一致的情况，如存在多种诊断标签，包括功能性障碍、神经官能症、神经症、疑病症、癔症、躯体化障碍等等。老百姓往往不能理解这些名词的意义，听到一个诊断名词就会认为自己多了一种疾病，会加重思想负担，造成病情迁延不愈。

二、疑难杂症与躯体化

当个体的压力大到以其智力想不出好的应对方式时，压力就会渗透到潜意识层面。而潜意识层面对压力的处置通常是转换，通过防御机制把压力改头换面，通过心理或生理的症状表现出来。这种处置的主要方式有两种：一种是用心理症状来表达压力，这些症状包括抑郁、焦虑、强迫、恐惧等；

另一种则是用生理症状来表达压力,称之为躯体化。

所谓躯体化,即有明显的躯体症状表现,但无肯定的或足够的病理证据,更多地可能与心理因素密切相关[4]。躯体化是一种症状,可见于许多疾病和障碍,如躯体疾病伴发的情绪障碍、心身综合征,常见的精神障碍即抑郁障碍、焦虑障碍、躯体症状障碍等。当这些患者以躯体化症状出现时,非心理精神科医生往往很难识别,造成很多所谓的疑难杂症,而其实质则是心身疾病。

三、躯体化症状的成因

(一)躯体症状表现受身与心共同影响

人是由躯体和心理共同组成的,人的躯体和心理是矛盾的统一体。医疗的对象是人,人不仅仅是一个生物体,有自然属性,而且还有社会属性,更有复杂的心理活动。既往研究表明,躯体症状的产生除与5-羟色胺系统和下丘脑-垂体-肾上腺轴这两个系统的基因变异有关外[5],同时还与精神心理因素密切相关。慢性压力可以引起自主神经活动增强。研究发现,暴露在慢性压力环境中,如生活在战争环境中,与躯体化症状的发生相关[6]。当机体处于焦虑或愤怒状态时,其肾上腺素、肾上腺皮质激素及抗利尿激素增加,可引起交感神经活动亢进,亢进的交感神经一方面引起心率增加、心输出量增加,另一方面导致末梢血管阻力增加,两者共同作用于机体,最终导致血压上升。类似地,当精神因素作用于大脑引起交感神经和副交感神经活动亢进时,亢进的副交感神经可导致胃酸分泌增多,同时亢进的交感神经导致胃黏液分泌减少,破坏性因素的增加与保护性因素的减少,最终引起消化性溃疡,出现胃痛、反酸、嗳气等症状。

(二)躯体化症状的理论解释

1. 心理动力学理论

当成人在遇到人际冲突、压抑、应激、创伤等压力时,婴幼儿期对外界刺激的躯体反应就会重现,借此可将自己的内心矛盾或冲突转换成躯体不适,表现出各种疾病的生理症状,从而摆脱自我的困境。Freud把这一过程叫作"再躯体化",它是一个退化过程[7]。事实上精神分析的观点认为,冲突是个体生活固有的一部分[8]。冲突的产生导致了焦虑,引起神经系统功能改变,最终引起脆弱器官的病变,出现那些不能解释的躯体症状,以此作为对自身内部和(或)外部环境恐惧的替代,并通过这种变相的发泄来缓解情绪上的冲突和矛盾[9]。

2. 心理生理学理论

该理论研究侧重于心身疾病的发病过程,重点说明哪些心理社会因素,通过何种生物学机制(包括心理神经中介途径、心理神经内分泌途径、心理神经免疫学途径)作用于何种状态的个体,导致何种疾病的发生。

3. 认识理论

该理论认为,神经质的人格特征、不良心境影响认知过程,一方面使当事人对躯体信息的感觉增强,选择性注意于躯体感觉;另一方面还使当事人用躯体疾病来解释上述感觉的倾向加强,助长与疾病有关的联想和记忆,及对自身健康的负性评价[10]。患者常常因为其症状不能得到正确的诊治而反复求医,从而导致情感沮丧、回避及社会功能受损,最终形成新的压力来源。我们可以将其称之为认知-知觉模型。患者之所以发病则是认知-知觉模型出现了障碍。

4. 行为学习理论

该理论源自米勒(Miller)提出的"内脏学习"的理论——疾病可以通过学习而获得[11]。行为学习理论认为,当某些社会环境刺激引发个体习得性心理和生理反应时,由于个体素质上的或特殊环境因素的强化,或通过泛化作用,使得这些习得性心理和生理反应被固定下来,最终演变成为症状和疾病。

5. 综合发病机制

针对某一个具体的患者,我们不能拘泥于某一理论,而是应综合各种理论,互相补充,形成综合的心身疾病发病机制理论,才能更好地解释临床患者的表现。

四、识别与处理

(一)诊断原则

这类患者有一个共同的特点,即"病在身,根在心"。但由于综合医院普通科室医生对心身医学和心身疾病的认识和了解仍存在不足,且大多数患者又拒绝因躯体症状就诊于心理科或精神科,以致其诊断困难。诊断此类症状应掌握以下几个原则:① 疾病的发生包括心理、社会因素,明确其与躯体症状的时间关系;② 躯体症状是否有明确的器质性病理改变,或存在已知的病理生理学变化;③ 排除可能的精神疾病。

(二)治疗原则——心身同治

心身疾病的治疗原则除了以解除症状为目标的一般内科躯体治疗以外,还需要有以减少复发、维持疗效稳定为目标的心理、社会治疗,帮助病人良好应对处理疾病过程中的有关心理、社会问题,最低限度地减少心理、社会因素的影响。故而,心身疾病的治疗有三个目标,即:消除心理社会刺激因素;消除心理学病因;消除生物学症状。

此类疾病治疗难度较大,需要患者同时具有"三心",即治疗疾病的信心、下定用药的决心及等待疗效的耐心。因此,我们给出以下建议:① 及早考虑心身疾病的可能,并将诊断告知患者;② 尽量让患者看一个医生,尽可能减少患者与其他医务人员接触;③ 确定心理、社会诱因,但要避免牵强附会;④ 安排定期门诊,但要间隔2~6周;⑤ 制订计划(如列出主要问题,逐一解决);⑥ 仅对客观发现做进一步检查,而对主观不适主诉采取忽略;⑦ 避免轻率下诊断,避免诊断反复和自相矛盾;⑧ 不要治疗患者并不存在的问题;⑨ 对患者产生的症状尽量使用解释模式;⑩ 对治疗效果不佳者建议精神科会诊。

（三）预防原则

此类症状预防原则主要包括：心身同治、从早做起（从小做起）、健全人格、矫正行为、消除刺激、积极疏导。

预防此类疾病，我们建议平时生活中应该学做三件事：学会关门——学会关紧昨天和明天这两扇门，过好每一个今天，每一个今天过得好就是一辈子过得好；学会计算——即学会计算自己的幸福和计算自己做对的事情。计算幸福会使自己越计算越幸福，计算做对的事情会使自己越计算越对自己有信心；学会放弃——特别推荐汉语中一个非常好的词，就是"舍得"。记住，是"舍"在先，"得"在后，世界上的事情总是有"舍"才有"得"。同时还要学说三句话："算了！"——即指对于一个无法改变的事实的最好办法就是接受这个事实；"不要紧！"——即不管发生什么事情，哪怕是天大的事情，也要对自己说："不要紧"！记住，积极乐观的态度是解决任何问题和战胜任何困难的第一步；"会过去的！"——不管雨下得多么大，连续下了多少天也不停，你都要对天会放晴充满信心，因为天不会总是阴的。自然界是这样，生活也是这样。只要我们平时能学会做好这三件事、学会说这三句话，我们的心情就能保持快乐。

五、总结

临床上的所谓疑难杂症中，约1/3的患者存在心理精神问题。虽然医生有必要确定疾病的生理基础，但因为几乎所有的躯体疾病都存在心理因素的影响，而这些精神心理因素往往又决定了疾病发病、临床表现、持续时间以及对治疗的敏感性，故而，作为一个医生应认识和掌握心身医学知识，从而识别并减少临床上的疑难杂症。

迄今为止，心身疾病的相关研究仍较为缺乏，心身疾病的发病机制与临床研究必将大有作为。

参考文献

[1] Kroenke K，Spitzer RL，Williams JB，et al. Physical symptoms in primary care. Predictors of psychiatric disorders and functional impairment [J]. Arch Fam Med，1994，3(9)：774 - 779.

[2] Fava A. The concept of psychosomatic disorder [J]. Psychother Psychosom，1992，58(1)：1 - 12.

[3] 吴文源. 持续的躯体形式疼痛障碍患者抑郁症状的特征及治疗[J]. 中国心理卫生杂志，2003，17(3)：147 - 149.

[4] 美国精神医学学会编著. 精神障碍诊断与统计手册[M]. 北京：北京大学出版社，2005：301.

[5] Hollidays KL，Macfarlane GJ. Genetic variation in neuroendocrine genes associates with somatic symptoms in the general population：Results from the EPIFUND study [J]. J Psychosom Res，2010，68(5)：469 - 474.

[6] Hasic S，Kisoljakovic E，Jaclric R，et al. Influence of long term stress exposure on somatization symptoms outcome [J]. Bosn J Basic Med Sci，2004，4(1)：28 - 31.

[7] 弗洛伊德. 精神分析引论[M]. 北京：商务印书馆，1997：270 - 286.

[8] Carver CS，Scheier MF. 人格心理学[M]. 5 版. 上海：上海人民出版社，2011：191 - 193.

[9] 常桂花，孔伶俐，刘春文. 躯体形式障碍的病因学研究进展[J]. 国际精神病学杂志，2013，40(1)：46 - 48.

[10] Katon W. Depression and somatization：a review [J]. Am J Med，1982，72(3)：241 - 247.

[11] Miller GA. The Science of the Word [M]. Scientific American Library，1991：147.

[作者及发表刊物：

袁勇贵，刘晓云，陈素珍，牟晓冬. 临床上的疑难杂症与心身疾病[J]. 实用老年医学，2016，30(9)：708 - 711.]

平衡心理治疗与心身相关障碍

摘要： 心身相关障碍是一种失衡状态，针对这种失衡状态，我们在整合了多种心理治疗流派的治疗取向的基础上提出了平衡心理治疗（BPT）。BPT可分为团体治疗、个体治疗和家族治疗三种类型。就团体BPT而言，通过六个步骤的操作流程（奠基石、领悟会、症状析、心得志、放松术和互助谈）帮助患者打通思维之路的阻塞，帮助其平衡好"度"的掌握与"关系"的协调，同时实现身与心，个人、家庭与社会、自然的和谐统一，使个体保持积极、向上的平衡心理，从容地面对生活，达到最终治疗目标。

关键词： 平衡心理治疗；心身相关障碍；度；关系

平衡心理治疗（Balancing Psychotherapy, BPT）是一种建立在东方哲学体系之上，整合了精神分析、认知疗法、行为疗法、叙事治疗以及积极心理学等多种心理治疗流派的治疗取向。它运用平衡学的相关理论，紧紧围绕"度"和"关系"两个核心内容，来帮助个体实现心身平衡状态。正确运用BPT有利于心身疾病患者的心身康复以及生存质量的提高[1]。

一、心身相关障碍是一种失衡状态

心身相关障碍产生的根源在于个体潜意识中的矛盾冲突，当这种矛盾冲突积聚到一定程度后就会突破原来的平衡状态，表现出各种各样的症状来，如抑郁、焦虑、躯体化等[2]，使得个体更痛苦。而事实上，人生不如意常八九，人的一生，相当一部分时间，就是用来化解这些"不如意"，即不平衡的。个人对不平衡的处理不当，是烦恼甚至疾病的根源。

人不可能没有烦恼，喜或怒其实都是正常现象，关键在于能否做到"发而皆中节"。如果过了度，或狂喜，或至哀，那就是心态失衡甚至严重失衡了。一种情绪走了极端,就会排挤其他情感,例如范进中举,其情绪从中举前的"万念俱灰"到中举后的"欣喜若狂",每一个阶段都存在着某种情感严重超出了其应该所占据的分量,使得内稳态失衡,最终导致心理问题甚至疾病出现。

喜、怒、忧、思、悲、恐、惊等情绪的"不节"是中医认为的内在病因,也就是说各种情绪的不平衡会导致疾病。而五行学说认为,五脏对应着五种主要的情绪,而且这些情绪之间也是相生相克的。肝对应的情绪为怒,怒伤肝,悲胜怒;心对应的情绪为喜,喜伤心,恐胜喜;脾对应的情绪为思,思伤脾,怒胜思;肺对应的情绪为忧,忧伤肺,喜胜忧;肾对应的情绪为恐,恐伤肾,思胜恐(《内经·五运行大论》)。范进中举后过分喜悦兴奋,以至于一时精神失常,后来有人建议找一个范进平时最怕的人,打他一个嘴巴,并斥责他,之后范进就正常了。这就是五行学说所谓的"喜伤心,恐胜喜"。弗洛伊德精神分析实践中早已发现,抑郁者往往压抑了自己的愤怒,而以抑郁替代了愤怒,这颇类似于"悲胜怒";心理治疗师也常常能见到,有些焦虑者变得易怒,用愤怒压抑焦虑,这就是"怒胜喜"。可以看出其实这七种情绪是相生相克的,它们之间处于一种动态平衡[3-4]

二、平衡的表现和本质

平衡是一个相对概念,属于哲学范畴。平衡既是宇宙规律,也是社会规律。我们可以把平衡定义归纳为四个字[5]:(1)动:平衡不是一潭死水,是动态的(以蓄水池为例,它是有进水和出水的);(2)变:当平衡的一边改变时,另一边也会随之改变;(3)等:平衡中得到的和失去的总保持相等。好像进水总等于出水,才能保持水面高度不变;(4)定:保持平衡的特点就是平稳,总保持稳定。而其中"动"和"变"是平衡的表现,"等"和"定"是平衡的本质。

三、平衡的基本功能

平衡的基本功能有二:一是"度"的掌握,二是"关系"的协调。"度"掌握好了,事物呈平衡状态;"关系"协调好了,事物亦呈平衡状态。

(一) 度的掌握

度就是限度。客观规律显示:人类的任何活动都有个度的掌握问题,不到度,事不成;过了度,事变样。孔子所说的"过犹不及"即是很好的例证。"过犹不及"之所以成为千古名言,是因为它阐明了一条重要的平衡规律,这条规律指导人们的一切行动。

度的掌握涉及智慧、气质和品德问题,只有认识到度的重要性,认真在生活中掌握度,才可能避免许多麻烦。孔子提倡饮酒有度,食姜有度,批评学生有度(如批评子路),待人有度("温而厉"、"威而不猛"、"恭而安"),自我修养有度("毋意、毋必、毋固、毋我")。

(二) 关系的协调

这里所说的关系,指的是人与人、事与事、人与事之间互相作用、互相影响。关系的协调是人类行为中的一个重要内容。其中,根本的协调是人际关系的协调。

中国儒家的伦理学,主要就是讲关系的协调。日本作家井上靖在其所著《孔子》中有这样的表述:"'仁',人旁从二。无论是父子、主从、萍水相逢的旅伴,在两人中必然存在着双方都必须遵守的规矩,这就是'仁',用其他语言来表达,就是'关照','设身处地为他人着想'。"

总之,平衡术的基本功能就是度的掌握和关系的协调。从"度"来讲,适度就是平衡;从"关系"来讲,和谐共处就是平衡[2]。

四、平衡的四个层次

平衡从病因学角度来看,从宏观到微观,平衡可分为四个层次:

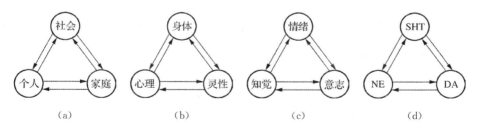

图1　平衡的四个层次

注:5-HT:5-羟色胺;NE:去甲肾上腺素;DA:多巴胺

（一）第一层次的平衡：个人-家庭-社会的平衡

当一个人的心理处于平衡状态，就会体现一个人在社会活动中躯体健康、思维敏捷、反应灵活、情感表达恰如其分。家庭是由个人组成的，它不仅承载着人类的繁衍生存，更满足了两性之间的心理和生理需求。家庭成员间需要互相尊重、互相支持、互相理解，共同承担家庭重任[1]。社会是发展进步只有顺其自然，与时俱进，才能在激烈竞争的社会中生存和发展，这是生物进化的普遍规律。家庭又是社会的基本构成单元，一个好的社会环境又会促进个人和家庭的发展，从而达到一个稳定的状态。

（二）第二层次的平衡：身心灵的平衡

其中，身指躯体（意识）；心指心理，主要指情绪（潜意识）；灵主要指精神和灵性状态（系统），如对生命意义价值的思考，以及人的生死观、苦乐观等。作为一个整体，身心灵包含了两层含义，一是指"身、心、灵"三个层面，即从三个不同层面去理解；二是指三者的整合体，即三者之间的互动关系，旨在促进"身、心、灵"三者之间关系的良性发展，进而实现全人类的健康[6]。身的活动离不开心，心的运作主要体现在知情意，灵的运作可表现于宗教信仰的灵修活动中[7]。

灵性的修炼就是自我的融合，即个体的小我和宇宙的大我的融合，也就是天人合一。通过这种融合性的修炼，我们可以获得内在的力量，深刻的反省自我，把智慧的光芒投射到我们的内在，从而提高自身的层次[8]。目前关于身心灵修养的方式主要在瑜伽、催眠、气功、中医养生等方面，特别是催眠术与瑜伽，更是风靡全球[9]。

（三）第三层次平衡：知情意的平衡

知情意的三角平衡是心理健康的标准。知就是认知，包括感知觉、思维；情就是情感情绪；意是意志行为。如果个体的知情意不平衡，那心理问题可能就出现了。

（四）第四层次的平衡：单胺递质的平衡

微观层面上，经典的单胺假说仍是我们解释心身（心理）疾病的发病和治疗机制的关键理论。如抑郁等的产生与血清中去甲肾上腺素(NE)、5-羟色胺(5-HT)和多巴胺(DA)水平的失衡等因素密切相关[9]。尽管该假说遭到质疑,但可以说即使其不是源头,也一定是中间某个步骤。

前述四个层次从宏观到微观对平衡进行了详细的阐述,这四个层次之间也是相互联系和相互制约的,任何一个层次的平衡被打破,必然会影响其他层次的平衡。另外,从治疗学角度来看,目前的治疗手段,不论是药物治疗、物理治疗,还是心理治疗,都是通过调节微观环境中的单胺递质平衡的失调入手的,逐渐达到第三、第二和第一层次的平衡。

五、BPT 简介

BPT 就是运用心身平衡理论和方法打通思维之路的阻塞,帮助来访者平衡好"度"的掌握与"关系"的协调。首先,通过分析病因,找到思维之路阻塞内稳态失衡的原因,然后再引导病人从本质和全局上对所遇到的问题进行认识,并举出相应的事例加以比较,让病人能够站在另一个角度审视自我,深化对自己问题的认知,最后与其一起探讨如何清除阻塞,并充分发挥病人的主观能动性,来激发、调动机体的物质能量,促进机体病理状态的良性转归,重建心身平衡。生理学奖得主伊丽莎白等总结出的长寿之道是[10]:人要活百岁,合理膳食占 25%,其他占 25%,而心理平衡的作用占到了 50%。

BPT 寻求传统的病理心理治疗与当代流行的积极心理治疗的完美融合,强调在不同的文化背景下,纵析时间线,实现心身的多维度平衡,即不仅仅要关注此时此地的当下,还要清晰理解过去的个体经历,更要面向未来。

BPT 的适应证包括心身相关障碍(如心身症状障碍、心身疾病、躯体疾病伴发心身症状等)、躯体症状障碍、抑郁障碍、焦虑障碍、失眠症及各类心理问题。

六、BPT 的治疗目标

BPT 指导个体的心理来适应家庭、社会、生态环境,特别是对生存环境产生的不良刺激,使个体能够及时有效地通过自我调节达到心身平衡[11]。

其治疗目标是实现身与心、个人、家庭与社会、自然的和谐统一，是个体达到积极的、向上的平衡心理，从容地面对生活。

七、BPT 的治疗步骤

平衡心理治疗可分为团体治疗、个体治疗和家庭治疗三种类型，每种类型大致包括六个步骤的操作流程，但这六个步骤的顺序并非固定不变，是可以相互融通，动态调整的。

（一）平衡奠基石

建立信任关系；治疗关系建立时的破冰效应；了解基本情况。病人的信任，来访者自愿原则是建立良好医患关系的基础，是一个疗法是否能见效不可或缺的根本。

（二）平衡领悟会

情绪情感是人们对客观事物是否符合自身需要的态度的体验，是与人的社会性需要相联系的主观体验。情感平衡是心理幸福感的重要组成部分，是一个人根据自己选择的标准对其生活质量所做的总体评价[12]。情绪驱使我们采取行动（如逃避、面对或宣泄），表达情绪，譬如哭泣或大笑都可以释放紧张和压力，任由情绪缘由的能量自然地流动与消耗，可以更好地帮助寻找症状的成因。通过导入 BPT 的核心理论，即"度的掌握"和"关系的协调"，以及讲故事（成功案例、哲理故事）、解读平衡箴言，启发来访者领悟自己心理问题的症结所在。

（三）平衡症状析

具体分析，剖析失衡原因，提高患者自信。平衡式的人生主要包括六个方面：家庭、事业、财富、朋友、健康和成长。六个方面都很重要，缺少任何一方面，都可能导致身心的失衡。

（四）平衡心得志

无论你是为了考试而复习，还是为了减肥而锻炼，有一点是共同的：必须进行有效的训练，包括一系列有效的重复动作和循序渐进的努力。心理训练也是如此,患者需要完成家庭作业,填写平衡反馈单,包括建立治疗目标,梳理治疗心得,加深自我分析,表达治疗信心等内容。"目标"能激发生命活力,也有助于我们思绪的整理[10]。而目标的实现无疑会让人非常快乐,但实现不了就会使来访者受挫,对治疗丧失信心。故此这里要注意:"目标"一定要切实可行,不宜过大,小步子原则,逐一实现为宜,否则会起副作用。

(五)平衡放松术

不同的来访者最适合的放松术可能不一样,是因人而异的。一般包括动态与静态两部分。

1. 动态放松术

包括太极拳、瑜伽、平衡保健操等。

① 太极拳:宋代周敦颐《太极图说》记载[13]:"太极动而生阳,动极而静,静而生阴。阴极复动,一动一静,互为其根,分阴分阳,两仪立焉。五行——阴阳也,阴阳——太极也。太极本无极也。五行之生也,各一其性。无极之真,二五之精,妙合而凝。乾道成男,坤道成女。两气交感,生化万物,万物生生而变化无穷焉。"太极拳动作体松圆活,快慢适度,分清虚实。打拳时按套路调整身体的姿势,进行招式动作,是练形。通过守意,使意念归一,排除杂念,调整心理活动,清静养神。

② 瑜伽:通过瑜伽训练不仅使人以新的境界回归本我,而且还能使人感悟自我、领悟超我。从古至今,瑜伽都特别强调发展人际情谊、促进和谐,而且要求彻底冲破种族、年龄、性别、宗教和信仰等限制,追求人类的博爱和平等,这种基本理念使瑜伽自始至终坚持非常明确的练习目标,即让人们从一切精神怨恨以及与之关联的各种精神心理和生理疾病中解脱出来,达到最佳的和谐与超脱状态[14]。

③ 平衡保健操:通过平衡保健操的适宜性训练,能够增强体质,同时有助于改善全身关节滑利、软组织的血液循环和神经体液的调节,活跃肌肉及软组织的营养代谢,起到放松痉挛肌肉、牵引挛缩肌腱和韧带,提高和恢复身体软组织及各关节的活动能力。

2. 静态放松术

包括生物反馈训练、听息、冥想、自我催眠等。

杯子里的水是浑浊的,静的时候才能看到灰尘。所以环境静下来了,人的杂念反而"增多"了,这其实不是说杂念增多了而是嘈杂时候烦劳的人们往往注意不到。所以,"静"是平衡放松术中相当重要的一面,入静不是简单意义上的什么都不想,而是一种专注的状态。譬如听息,就是听自己呼吸之气,意念专注于呼吸之间(呼吸之间的停顿为息,功力越高的人越长),开始练习时只用耳听,感受一呼一吸即可,至于呼吸的快慢、粗细浅深,皆任其自然变化,不用意识去支配它。渐渐的杂念就沉淀了,听到后来神气合一,杂念全无[15],而后当忘记呼吸的时候内心会变得清明,此时五感清晰,外面的干扰如映照在镜子中的影像,过后不留痕迹。

① 生物反馈训练:生物反馈是 20 世纪 60 年代发展起来的一门技术,它利用操作性条件反射原理,使主体得以了解原本很难意识到的机体变化,并通过学习达到随意控制和矫正不正常生理变化的目的[16]。有研究证实,生物反馈训练能有效改善个体的心理问题[17]。

② 听息:"听息"出自《庄子·人间世》,其要旨是:心随于息,息随于心;心息相依,绵绵密密。孔子说:"你专一心志,不要用耳去听,而要用心去听;不要用心去听,而要用气去听。用耳去听,只能听到耳所能听到的声音;用心去听,只能听到与心相合的食物。气这个东西,是空虚而能接纳一切事物的。唯有'虚'才能把'道'聚集起来"[18]。

③ 冥想:关于"冥想",从认知角度可认为"冥想是通过身心的自我调节,建立特殊的注意机制,最终影响个体的心理过程的一系列联系"[19];从行为角度指出冥想"是包括身体放松、呼吸调节、注意聚焦三个阶段的综合过程"[20];从心理体验角度强调冥想可以"通过自我调控练习,让个体产生一种心理幸福感"[21]。因此我们可以说,冥想不仅强调身体放松,也强调认知和心理放松,是一种综合性的心理和行为训练。

④ 自我催眠:刘凌[22]在《潜意识与催眠术》中,提出催眠的实质即如何通过暗示来影响被催眠者的潜意识。通过对潜意识的积极暗示,可以充分调动人们的潜能,创造超乎想象的奇迹。徐静[23]也在《浅析催眠术与催眠疗法》中指出催眠治疗不仅具有广度而且具有深度,是走入潜意识深处的一条

捷径,也是个体认知自我的一扇窗口。

(六) 平衡互助谈

发挥团体治疗的优势。欧文亚隆认为心理治疗的疗效在团体治疗中可得到更好的体验[24]。心身疾病患者团体成员和团体环境间有着丰富而微妙的动力学互助成员会塑造自己的社会缩影,会逐个吸纳每个人特有的防御行为。团体互动越自发,社会缩影的发展就越快速真实,团体成员中主要的问题被引出、讨论、解决的可能性就越大[25]。

八、小结

心身相关障碍是一类与心理社会因素有着密切关系的躯体疾病。在这类患者中,心理社会因素可以是疾病发生的原因之一,也可以是疾病发展的促进因素。对于这类患者的治疗,须兼顾心理和生理两个方面平衡的调整,才能取得满意效果,达到有效控制症状的根本目的。平衡心理治疗从"度的掌握"和"关系的协调"两个方面入手,对心身相关障碍患者心身症状的成因进行深入剖析,通过纠正不正确的认知信念和导入积极的行为方式,减少患者的烦恼,改变患者的心身症状,最终达到治疗患者的目的。

参考文献

[1] 王文远. 中国平衡心理学理论研究[J]. 前进论坛(健康中华),2006(1):37-39.

[2] 葛楚英. 平衡——人类生存之路[M]. 湖北:湖北人民出版社,2006.

[3] 吕爱平. 论中医辩证思维的内涵与特点[J]. 中国中医基础医学杂志,2009,(7):481.

[4] 盛国光. "和"之为义及其在中医学中的体现[J]. 中医杂志,2006,47(6):410-411.

[5] 葛楚英. 平衡学[M]. 湖北:湖北人民出版社,2013.

[6] 陈丽云. 身心灵全人类模式—中国文化与团体心理辅导[M]. 北京:中国轻工业出版社,2009.

[7] 傅佩荣. 心灵导师—身心灵整合之道[M]. 上海:上海三联书店,2009.

[8] 周慧虹. 太极身心灵修炼及其和谐价值研究[D]. 湖南师范大学硕士学位论文,2012.

[9] 吕静静.稳心颗粒联合米氮平对抑郁症及血清 NE、5-HT 和 DA 的影响[D]. 河北：河北医科大学硕士学位论文,2012.

[10] 李宏磊.心理因素或决定寿命长短[N]. 新华每日电讯,2014-8-8(10).

[11] 王文远.中国平衡心理学理论研究[J].前进论坛(健康中华),2006(1):37 - 39.

[12] 梁瑞华,毛富强,赵朋,等.内观认知疗法对大学生心理因素的影响研究:情感平衡、领悟社会支持和容纳他人[J].中国行为医学科学,2008,17(12):1106 - 1108.

[13] 杨全祥.太极拳拳学思想的理论渊源与基本意蕴[J].河南社会科学,2007(5):5.

[14] 单清华,刘莹,王振涛,等.瑜伽文化足迹及现代健身价值研究[J].体育与科学,2009,30(5):46 - 48.

[15] 天心见.用精神守护生命——道家养生法精粹(续)[J].中华养生保健(上半月),2002(6):19 - 20.

[16] 郑延平.生物反馈仪的临床实践[J].北京:高等教育出版社,2003.

[17] 陈艳红,陈幼平,李丹,等.生物反馈训练对大学生心理健康的影响[J].中国健康心理学杂志,2013,21(12):1831 - 1833.

[18] 金志良.听息、止观和坐忘[J].气功杂志,1998(9):486.

[19] Cahn BR, Polich J. Meditation states and traits: EEG, ERP and neuroimaging studies[J]. Psychological Bulletin,132(2):180 - 211.

[20] 姜镇英.冥想训练对美国中学游泳选手训练后的焦虑、心境状态及心率恢复的影响[J].体育科学,2000,20(6):66 - 74.

[21] Walsh R, Shapiro SL. The meeting of meditation disciplines and Western psychology: A mutually enriching dialogue[J]. American Psychologist,2006(61):227 - 239.

[22] 刘凌.潜意识与催眠术[J].湘潮(下半月)(理论),2007(9):41 - 42.

[23] 徐静.浅析催眠术与催眠疗法[J].法制与社会,2008(34):368 - 369.

[24] 欧文·亚隆.团体心理治疗—理论与实践(第五版)[M].北京:中国轻工业出版社,2010.

[25] 杨莉萍,张秀敏.社会建构论语境中的团体心理治疗[J].医学与哲学,2013,34(1):47 - 49.

[作者及发表刊物：

袁勇贵,黄河,张玲俐,王彩云,刘晓云,徐治,张文瑄.平衡心理治疗与心身相关障碍[J].实用老年医学,2017,31(10):906 - 909.]

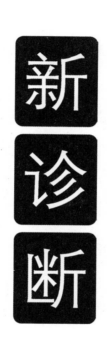

心身症状障碍

摘要：根据综合性医院医生的实际需求出发，我们创新性地提出了"心身症状障碍"的疾病诊断标准和症状严重度评定标准。心身症状障碍是一种新的疾病诊断，它不同于神经症性障碍、躯体症状障碍、心身疾病和躯体疾病伴发心身症状等疾病，应注意与之鉴别诊断。它的提出有效解决了综合科临床医生的困惑，有利于指导这类患者的临床治疗，丰富了心身相关障碍分类体系的内容，并能有效规避《精神卫生法》对非精神科医师的限制。

关键词：心身症状障碍；诊断；鉴别诊断

一、心身症状障碍的提出

在综合性医院，临床上常见这样一组人群，存在焦虑、抑郁、疼痛、失眠和躯体化等症状，他们未达到目前已知的所有精神障碍诊断标准，但是这些症状的存在已经严重影响到了他们的日常工作和生活。对于达不到诊断标准的情况该如何下诊断？这给临床医生带来了困惑和难题。这就要求我们给这类患者提供一个新的诊断。中华医学会心身医学分会的临床专家们经临床研究后提出了"心身症状障碍"的诊断。

二、定义与诊断标准

1. 心身症状障碍的定义

一组与急、慢性心理社会因素密切相关的综合征，病人具有一定的人格基础，主要表现为焦虑、抑郁、失眠、疼痛、躯体化症状等症状中的一种或几种症状。症状没有可证实的器质性病变作基础，或虽存在一定的躯体疾病，但疾病的严重程度与病人的症状严重程度不相称，病人感到痛苦和无能为力，自知力不全。不符合现有的精神障碍的诊断标准。

2. 心身症状障碍的诊断标准

心身症状障碍需符合下列四个标准：

症状标准(至少有下列一项)：① 抑郁；② 焦虑；③ 失眠；④ 疼痛；⑤ 其他躯体化症状等。

严重标准：社会功能部分受损或自感痛苦,促使其主动求医。

病程标准：1周以上。

排除标准：排除现有的各类精神障碍。

3. 心身症状障碍严重度的评定(见表1)

表1 心身症状障碍严重度评定量表

条目	评分
应激	0无；1轻度；2中度；3重度
严重度	0无影响；1轻度影响日常生活和工作；2中度影响日常生活和工作；3不能正常生活和工作
病程	0一周以内；1一个月内；2三个月内；3三个月以上

临床医生可根据表1的评定结果,给出具体的建议：轻度(0～3分)：可以自我调节；中度(4～6分)：建议心身科门诊就诊；重度(7～9分)：建议心身科住院治疗或精神科治疗。

三、心身症状障碍的鉴别诊断

心身症状障碍是一种新的疾病诊断,它不同于以前的神经症性障碍、躯体症状障碍、心身疾病和躯体疾病所致心身症状等疾病。

1. 心身症状障碍与神经症性障碍的比较(见表2)

表2 心身症状障碍与神经症性障碍比较

	心身症状障碍	神经症
心理社会因素	病因	诱因
人格特征	A 型行为、D 型行为	神经质
伴发躯体疾病	可以伴发	常不伴发
病程	大多3个月以内	3个月以上
症状	较轻	较重

	心身症状障碍	神经症
核心症状	躯体化症状＋心理症状	心理症状＋躯体化症状
治疗	心身干预治疗(药物＋心理)	综合性治疗(心理＋药物)
预后	轻度较好,中重度较差	较差

2. 心身症状障碍与躯体症状障碍比较(见表3)

表3　心身症状障碍与躯体症状障碍比较

	心身症状障碍	躯体症状障碍
临床表现	常为焦虑、抑郁、失眠等	一个或多个躯体症状
先占观念	常无	过度的想法、感受或行为;或与健康相关的过度担心
病程	≥1周	≥6个月
严重程度	轻、中度	中、重度
治疗	心理治疗或药物治疗	药物治疗＋心理治疗
预后	较好	较差或差

3. 心身反应、心身症状障碍和心身疾病的比较(见表4)

表4　心身反应、心身症状障碍与心身疾病比较

	心身反应	心身症状障碍	心身疾病
心理社会因素	常为急性	常为急性或亚急性	少数为急性重大应激,多为慢性应激
人格特征	A型行为	A型行为、D型行为	A型行为、D型行为、述情障碍
器质性病变	无	常无	有
病程	短,1～2周	大多3个月以内	3个月以上
症状	轻	中	重
治疗	心理治疗为主	轻度:心理治疗 中重度:心理治疗＋(精神)药物治疗	心理治疗＋(精神)药物治疗＋物理治疗
预后	好	较好	较差
转化	可转为心身症状障碍	可转为与心身疾病共患	可与心身症状障碍共患

4. 心身症状障碍与躯体疾病伴发心身症状的鉴别(见表5)

表5　心身症状障碍与躯体疾病伴发心身症状比较

	心身症状障碍	躯体疾病所致心身症状
临床表现	常为焦虑、抑郁、失眠等	焦虑、抑郁等症状
病因	生活事件	躯体疾病
病程	≥1周	即时
严重程度	轻、中度	与躯体疾病有关
治疗	心理治疗或药物治疗	躯体治疗＋药物治疗＋心理治疗
预后	较好	与躯体疾病有关

四、心身症状障碍诊断的意义

1. 解决了临床医生的困惑

心身症状障碍的提出,让综合医院的临床医生有了诊断的依据,不再为这类疾病和患者无处可归而烦恼,心身疾病临床各科医生都可诊治。

2. 有效指导这类患者的临床治疗

诊断是治疗的前提,有了专门的诊断,可以让我们更好地总结经验,更好地指导治疗。

3. 丰富了心身医学体系的内容

目前国际上尚未有一套完整的心身疾病分类和诊断体系,心身症状障碍的提出,对完善心身医学体系具有重要意义。

4. 有效规避了《精神卫生法》的限制

《精神卫生法》第二十九条明确规定:精神障碍的诊断应当由精神科执业医师作出。那么综合医院临床各科医生遇到这类患者怎么办呢? 就不能诊治而一定需要转精神科吗? 问题关键是这类患者大多数不愿转精神科,再加上这类患者约占综合医院门诊的1/3,精神科医生也忙不过来。因此,心身症状障碍属于心身疾病范畴,不属于精神障碍,它的提出,有效规避了《精神卫生法》的限制。

[作者:袁勇贵　吴爱勤]

健康焦虑障碍是否是一种新型焦虑障碍

摘要： 健康焦虑是一种连续性的症状谱,从轻微的健康关注到过度的健康担忧,其关注的健康问题集中在对未来的健康担忧上而非当前。近年来有人提出健康焦虑障碍(HAD)可能是一种新型的焦虑障碍,它具有独征的临床特征和认知模式。但 HAD 尚没有明确的诊断标准,它与疑病症或疾病焦虑障碍、躯体症状障碍、惊恐障碍、广泛性焦虑障碍、强迫症等的关系也需进一步明确。在未来的研究中,需进一步完善 HAD 的诊断标准,开展治疗预后和生物学特征的研究,以便证实其诊断地位。

关键词： 焦虑；认知模式；诊断标准

健康焦虑是指个体对当前身体健康状况或未来健康状况的过度担心[1]。健康焦虑在普通人群中的发生率达 5%[2],在综合性医疗机构就诊患者中将近 9%[3],恢复期患者达 30%～50%[2]。Sunderland 等[4]对澳大利亚人群调查发现,5.7% 的人在一生中某些时点患有健康焦虑;4.2% 的人在过去的 12 个月中经历过健康焦虑;3.4% 的人在调查时正经历着健康焦虑;健康焦虑的患病率似乎在中年时期达到高峰(7.4%),而到老年时期又下降了几乎一半。健康焦虑被认为是连续性的症状谱,一端是对健康的轻微关注,另一端则是对健康的过度关注[5]。有人认为严重的健康焦虑等同于美国精神障碍诊断与统计手册第 4 版(diagnostic and statistical manual of mental disorders Ⅳ,DSM-Ⅳ)中的疑病症,或美国精神障碍诊断与统计手册第 5 版(DSM-5)中疾病焦虑障碍(illness anxiety disorder,IAD)[6]。尽管 2012 年 Rachman 首次提出健康焦虑障碍(health anxiety disorders,HAD)这一概念,并认为 HAD 与惊恐障碍、社交恐惧、广泛性焦虑障碍一样,均属于焦虑障碍,是一种独立的疾病单元,但他并未对 HAD 的临床表现、生物学特征、治疗及疾病转归做进一步的详细研究,也未提出相应的诊断标准。因此,我们对这一问题作了初步探讨,以明确 HAD 的诊断地位。

一、HAD 具有独特的临床特征和认知模式

(一) 临床症状

HAD 患者对疾病恐惧的来源主要有三方面:自身经历严重或烦恼的事件,亲属或近友的重大事件和接收了威胁性的信息[1]。HAD 患者所具有的临床表现与其灾难化的认知密切相关,由于错误的健康认知,HAD 患者极易将正常的或轻微的躯体症状灾难化,从而表现出一系列特有的行为,如寻求保证、重复就诊、逃避行为等。

1. 侵入性想象

Salkovskis 等[7]通过两例疑病症患者的案例分析了健康焦虑患者侵入性想象这一行为,他们认为健康焦虑患者的侵入性想象类似于强迫症患者的强迫行为。比如文中列举的案例,患者因荨麻疹持续数月认为自己可能患有白血病,在医师和家人保证没有问题的情况下仍然有这种想法。值得注意的是,HAD 患者的侵入性想象关注的是未来的健康而非当下或过去,且侵入性想象和焦虑之间有相互恶化的作用。

2. 寻求保证

寻求保证是 HAD 患者安全行为中的一种,由于焦虑和侵入性想象的存在,患者会不断去医院就诊,以确定自己没有健康问题[8],然而科学的检查和医师的保证并不能让患者降低的焦虑程度持续很长时间,相反会加重保证之后的焦虑程度[7,9]。

3. 逃避行为

逃避也是一种安全行为,HAD 患者可因安全行为的不同而分为寻求保证型和逃避型。HAD 患者因为恐惧严重疾病的发生,所以选择不去医院、避免与疾病有关的场景等。逃避行为加重了患者的焦虑程度,甚至产生一系列强迫行为,比如因恐惧感染导致癌症而不断洗手。当然也有研究表明,

明智的安全行为有利于疾病的治疗[9]。

4. 躯体症状

HAD 患者往往存在一些正常的或轻微的躯体症状,这些症状的存在不仅加重了健康焦虑的程度,还会随焦虑程度加重而更加频繁。

(二) 认知模式

尽管 HAD 的研究逐渐增加,但是关注其认知的研究还少之又少。Salkovskis 和 Warwick 认为 HAD 的核心认知包括四部分,即:① 对即将和已有疾病可能性的感知;② 对疾病畏惧的感知;③ 对无法应对疾病的感知;④ 对不合理治疗资源的感知[10]。Marcus 等[11]研究健康焦虑患者后同样将 HAD 的认知归纳为四个方面:① 认为躯体症状十分危险;② 认为疾病不受控制;③ 认为自身疾病缺乏躯体症状;④ 认为恶劣的身体状况无法避免。比较而言,Salkovskis 和 Warwick 对 HAD 的认知概括更偏重于核心,这与其模式中健康焦虑患者持有的最重要的核心信念——紊乱的疾病相关信念一致[11]。而 Marcus 等[11]则是建立在个体的基础上,对大多数患者会出现的信念进行了总结概括。Taylor 和 Asmundson 则将认知因素(包括紊乱的信念和选择性记忆)、注意力因素和躯体感觉扩大化综合在一起,形成了健康焦虑的整合模型。有关 HAD 的认知模式多种多样,但重要的一点是,不同的模式都没有脱离对健康的焦虑和患者错误的扭曲的疾病认识。

值得注意的是,Salkovskis 和 Warwick 的 HAD 认知模式与 Clark 和 Barlow 的惊恐障碍认知模式相关[11]。惊恐障碍的认知模式涉及个体对躯体感觉和症状的灾难化误解,而强迫症的认知模式则表现为缺乏自信,总是不放心、怀疑、唯恐不合适,穷思竭虑,并与健康相关的恐惧联系在一起,这二者的认知模式在 HAD 认知模式的形成过程中起到了很大的促进作用[1]。在疑病症的认知行为模式中,对疾病灾难化的认知是极为重要的一个环节,因为灾难化的认知不仅给患者造成功能上的影响,还让患者时刻意识到疾病恐惧[12]。结合 HAD 的认知中有惊恐障碍的灾难化误解和强迫症中对疾病的怀疑、不放心,可以认为疑病症的认知模式与 HAD 的认知模式相同,只是在灾难化的程度上有所区别。

二、HAD 诊断标准的拟定

目前尚无 HAD 的诊断标准,但疑病症的诊断标准在 DSM 诊断体系中早已出现,并在 DSM-5 中改称 IAD。为了提高临床研究的一致性,结合多年的精神科临床工作经验和精神疾病诊断标准的结构模式,我们提出 HAD 的诊断标准,供临床医师验证。

1. 症状标准

(1)符合焦虑障碍的诊断标准。(2)对健康的侵入性想象关注于未来,而非当下或过去的健康状况。(3)有一种或多种躯体症状存在,如腹胀、心悸、便秘等。(4)存在反复寻求保证或逃避医疗保健的行为。

2. 严重标准

工作、生活受到影响。

3. 病程标准

符合症状标准至少已 3 个月。

4. 排除标准

排除 IAD(疑病症)、躯体化障碍、广泛性焦虑障碍、惊恐障碍、强迫症、恐惧症等。

三、与其他疾病的鉴别要点

健康焦虑障碍与其他疾病的鉴别诊断见表1。

1. 疑病症或 IAD

大多数的研究者认为,疑病症或 IAD 是 HAD 的一种极端形式,两者只是程度不同,而 Rachman[1] 和 Starcevic[6] 就疑病症的认知和概念提出了疑问。疑病症患者的信念是抵制不确定因素,关注当前和急性的危险因素,而健康焦虑患者是对未来可能的危险因素有所感知。同时疑病症是一个解剖术语(比如患者常常描述自己的腹部、肋骨下等解剖部位疼痛或不适),最终

表 1 健康焦虑障碍与其他疾病的鉴别诊断

疾病类型	患病率	严重程度	病程	对个体的影响	关注对象	歪曲信念和行为
健康焦虑障碍	5%[a]	由轻到重的症状谱	小于6个月	轻微或不影响	健康	可以控制
疾病焦虑障碍	1.3%~10%	伴躯体症状的疑病症	6个月	明显影响	疾病	无法控制
躯体症状障碍	高于1%	不伴躯体症状的疑病症	6个月	明显影响	躯体症状或疾病	可以控制或不可控制
疑病症	3%~9%	健康焦虑的极端形式	6个月	严重影响	疾病	无法控制
躯体化障碍	0.50%	轻中度	2年	轻度影响	躯体症状	可以控制
广泛性焦虑障碍	1.48‰	中度	6个月	轻度影响	未来	部分控制
惊恐障碍	男性1.3%，女性3.2%	发作时较重	1个月	发作时影响	躯体症状	无法控制
强迫症	0.3‰	中度	3个月	严重时影响	强迫观念	无法控制
恐惧症[b]	0.59‰	发作时较重	3个月	轻度影响	疾病	可以控制

疾病类型	躯体症状	先占观念	自我暗示	治疗的目的	治疗依从性	预后
健康焦虑障碍	不固定	无或轻微	轻微	消除症状	好	及时干预较好
疾病焦虑障碍	一般固定，也可涉及多个部位	严重	严重	消除症状或明确诊断	很差	很差
躯体症状障碍	不固定或固定	严重	轻度	消除症状或明确诊断	较差	较好/差
疑病症	固定	严重	严重	明确诊断	差	很差
躯体化障碍	不固定、多变	无或轻微	中度	消除症状	好	较好
广泛性焦虑障碍	可以有，可以控制	无或轻微	轻微	消除症状	较好	及时干预较好
惊恐障碍	突然发生，10 min达高峰，有濒死感	轻中度	轻微	消除症状	好	及时干预较好
强迫症	无	强迫观念	轻微	消除症状	较差	差
恐惧症[b]	不明显	轻微	轻微	消除症状	好	及时干预较好

注：a，为国外数据；b，指疾病恐惧，特定恐惧的一种

会归因于神经系统。此类患者反复就诊的目的是为了明确诊断,不愿意服药。Starcevic[6]认为疾病恐惧和疾病信念是疑病症的两种主要组成部分,健康焦虑和疑病症都有疾病恐惧的一部分特征(更精确地说,是与疾病相关的内容),而健康焦虑似乎没有疾病信念这一组成部分。但仔细地分析,可以发现疑病症与 IAD 之间还是具有稍许差别的,Starcevic[6]认为只有很少或没有躯体症状的患者才可以归为 IAD,这部分人大约占疑病症的 25%。由于界限划分并不很清晰,所以常常给临床诊断带来较大困难。

2. 躯体化障碍

患者以多种多样的、经常变化的躯体症状为主要表现,多为慢性波动性病程,常伴有社会、人际及家庭行为方面的问题。病程在 2 年以上,患者反复就诊的目的是为了减轻症状,愿意服药。而 HAD 具有歪曲的认知信念,以精神性焦虑为主。

3. 广泛性焦虑障碍

患者以缺乏明确对象和具体内容的提心吊胆和紧张不安为主要表现,很少诉说自身的躯体症状和对某些躯体感觉的误解[13]。而且广泛性焦虑患者伴有显著的自主神经症状、肌肉紧张及运动性不安。

4. 惊恐障碍

HAD 和惊恐障碍中的焦虑和恐惧都来自患者对躯体感觉灾难化的误解[14],但在临床表现和持续时间上仍有所区别。惊恐障碍患者的极度恐惧通常在持续 5～20 min 后逐渐平息,只剩下对健康的轻微焦虑,且惊恐的发作往往有特定的诱发因素或特殊的场所。而 HAD 的恐惧和焦虑持续存在,并且由于焦虑的持续性导致了患者对躯体感觉或某些轻微症状的高度警觉性。

5. 强迫症

HAD 与强迫症同属焦虑障碍,有研究表明两者都与抑郁有关[1],且两者侵入性和干扰性的想象在某些方面是相似的,只是 HAD 患者关注对健康的威胁以及恐惧严重疾病带来的后果[15]。重要的是,HAD 患者侵入性想象是与人格和个人经历有关的,而强迫症患者的这种想象通常与人格和个人经历不一致[7]。同时,强迫症患者知道自己的想象是不合理的并常常抵触,从而隐藏自己的行为,而 HAD 患者则是更多地倾向于寻求保证和帮助[16]。

6. 疾病恐惧症

疾病恐惧症是一种以过分和不合理地惧怕外界客体或处境(疾病)为主的恐惧症。如艾滋病恐惧症患者也会表现出疑病、焦虑、抑郁等症状,以往有明确的诱因,更多地认为是一种混合型神经症样障碍[17]。

四、HAD 的治疗现状

关于 HAD 的治疗目前尚没有系统的治疗研究,但以往的文献表明,认知行为疗法(cognitive behavioral therapy,CBT)治疗健康焦虑,无论其短期效果还是长期效果都非常明显[18]。而在药物治疗方面,对焦虑障碍治疗有效的选择性 5-羟色胺再摄取抑制剂可能对 HAD 治疗也有效[19],但是停药后药物的作用是否能够维持则不得而知。鉴于 HAD 患者主要表现为认知歪曲基础上的精神焦虑,建议在抗焦虑治疗的同时合并心理治疗,特别是治疗后期心理治疗应占主导地位。

五、展望

目前尚无足够证据证明 HAD 就是一种独立的焦虑障碍,尽管近年来焦虑障碍的发病机制有了一定的发展,但针对 HAD 的发病机制的研究较少,是否与 IAD 相似还是具有一种独特的发病机制,这一点单从其认知模式探讨是远远不够的。未来应该花更多的时间在认知模式的基础上探索其发病机制,如从神经心理学、神经生化学、神经电生理学、神经影像学、遗传学等多方面来寻找或证实 HAD 是否具有独特的生物学特征。另外,它的临床特征、诊治预后是否具有独特性也需时日去探讨证实。我们有理由相信,随着研究文献的逐渐增多,HAD 的诊断地位将会逐渐明确。

参考文献

[1] Rachman S. Health anxiety disorders: a cognitive construal[J]. Behav Res Ther, 2012,50(7/8):502-512.

[2] Fergus TA, Valentiner DP. Reexamining the domain of hypochondriasis: comparing the illness attitudes scale to other approaches[J]. J Anxiety Disord, 2009, 23 (6):760-766.

[3] Muse K, McManus F, Hackmann A, et al. Intrusive imagery in severe health anxiety: prevalence, nature and links with memories and maintenance cycles[J]. Behav Res Ther, 2010,48(8):792-798.

[4] Sunderland M, Newby JM, Andrews G. Health anxiety in Australia: prevalence, comorbidity, disability and service use [J]. Br J Psychiatry, 2013,202(1):56-61.

[5] Ferguson E. A taxometric analysis of health anxiety[J]. Psychol Med, 2009,39(2): 277-285.

[6] Starcevic V. Hypochondriasis and health anxiety: conceptual challenges[J]. Br J Psychiatry, 2013,202(1):7-8.

[7] Salkovskis PM, Warwick HM. Morbid preoccupations, health anxiety and reassurance: a cognitive-behavioural approach to hypochondriasis[J]. Behav Res Ther, 1986,24(5):597-602.

[8] Olatunji BO, Etzel EN, Tomarken AJ, et al. The effects of safety behaviors on health anxiety: an experimental investigation[J]. Behav Res Ther, 2011,49(11):719-728.

[9] Rachman S, Radomsky AS, Shafran R. Safety behaviour: a reconsideration[J]. Behav Res Ther, 2008,46(2):163-173.

[10] Hadjistavropoulos HD, Janzen JA, Kehler MD, et al. Core cognitions related to health anxiety in self-reported medical and non-medical samples[J]. J Behav Med, 2012,35(2):167-178.

[11] Marcus DK, Gurley JR, Marchi MM, et al. Cognitive and perceptual variables in hypochondriasis and health anxiety: a systematic review [J]. Clin Psychol Rev, 2007,27(2):127-139.

[12] Abramowitz JS, Deacon BJ, Valentiner DP. The short health anxiety inventory: psychometric properties and construct validity in a nonclinical sample[J]. Cogn Ther Res,2007,31(6):871 - 883.

[13] Marouf F, Giallourakis CC, Baer L, et al. Case records of the Massachusetts General Hospital. Case 33-2013. A 40-year-old woman with abdominal pain, weight loss, and anxiety about cancer[J]. N Engl J Med,2013,369(17):1639 - 1647.

[14] Clark DM. A cognitive approach to panic[J]. Behav Res Ther, 1986,24(4):461 - 470.

[15] Muse K, McManus F, Hackmann A, et al. Intrusive imagery in severe health anxiety: Prevalence, nature and links with memories and maintenance cycles[J]. Behav Res Ther,2010,48(8):792 - 798.

[16] Newth S, Rachman S. The concealment of obsessions[J]. Behav Res Ther,2001, 39(4):457 - 464.

[17] 王建平,王珊珊,蔺秀云,等. 艾滋病恐惧症的研究初探[J]. 心理科学进展,2004, 12(2):435 - 439.

[18] Seivewright H, Green J, Salkovskis P, et al. Cognitive-behavioural therapy for health anxiety in a genitourinary medicine clinic: randomised controlled trial[J]. Br J Psychiatry,2008,193(4):332 - 337.

[19] Abramowitz JS, Deacon BJ. Severe health anxiety:why it persists and how to treat it[J]. Compr Ther,2004,30(1):44 - 49.

[作者及发表刊物:

袁勇贵,张钰群. 健康焦虑障碍是否是一种新型焦虑障碍[J]. 中华脑科疾病与康复杂志(电子版),2015,5(2):70 - 73.(有改动)]

New opinion on the subtypes of poststroke depression in Chinese stroke survivors

Aim: Poststroke depression (PSD) is the most common complication of stroke. However, some stroke survivors with depression cannot meet the diagnostic criteria of PSD. The aim of this study was to propose the new conception of stroke patients with depression and then make them to receive reasonable diagnosis and treatment.

Methods: We first put forward the opinion that the general PSD should consist of PSD disorder (PSDD) and PSD symptoms (PS-DS) according to the *Diagnostic and Statistical Manual of Mental Disorder*-Fifth Edition (DSM-5) and ZhongDa diagnostic criteria-first edition (ZD-1), respectively. The ZD-1 was established based on the suggestions of 65 Chinese chief doctors considering that the symptoms of PSDS might be different from those of PSDD and the duration of DSM-5 was too strict. Then, 166 stroke inpatients were recruited, and the study was conducted using the diagnosis and classification of PSD to verify the new concept.

Results: A total of 24 (14.46%) and 80 (48.19%) stroke patients were diagnosed with PSDD and PSDS, respectively, according to individual diagnosis criteria. Moreover, patients meeting the diagnostic criteria of PSDD should satisfy the criteria of PSDS first. The distribution frequencies of depressive symptoms were different, which suggested that there might be discrepant depressive symptoms between PSDS and PSDD.

Conclusion: The present study proposes new opinion about the classification and diagnosis of depression in stroke survivors. The definition and criteria of PSDS are beneficial to explore phenomenological consistency and provide useful information for early recognition and appropriate interventions.

Keywords: poststroke depression, subtypes, diagnostic criteria

中 文 摘 要

中国卒中后抑郁分类的新视角

岳莹莹　刘　瑞　曹　音　吴岩峰　张石宁
李华杰　朱记军　姜文颢　吴爱勤　袁勇贵

目的：卒中后抑郁（post stroke depression，PSD）是脑卒中后的常见并发症，然而一些卒中伴发抑郁的患者并不能满足常规的 PSD 诊断标准。因此本研究旨在提出 PSD 分类并明确各类诊断标准，为 PSD 合理诊断和及时治疗提供理论依据。

方法：我们创新性的提出 PSD 分为卒中后抑郁症状障碍（post-stroke depressive symptoms disorder，PSDSD）和卒中后抑郁症（post-stroke depressive disorder，PSDD）并分别建立诊断标准，其中 PSDSD 的诊断标准是在已制定量表的基础上，依据 65 位中国副高级职称以上的神经及精神科医师的临床经验，并考虑 DSM-5 诊断 PSD 的局限性，参考精神疾病诊断模式建立 PSDSD 可操作性诊断标准，即 PSDS 中大诊断标准–第 1 版（ZhongDa diagnostic criteria of PSDS-first edition，ZD-1/PSDSD）；PSDD 的诊断则采用抑郁症（major depressive disorder，MDD）的诊断标准。然后收集 166 例卒中患者，对其进行 PSDSD 和 PSDD 诊断。

结果：在 166 例卒中患者中，按照 ZD-1/PSDSD 和 DSM-5 的标准分别有 80 例（48.19％）和 24 例（14.46％）患者被诊断为 PSDSD 和 PSDD，且诊断为 PSDD 的 24 例患者均满足 PSDSD 的诊断。但两类 PSD 患者的抑郁症状分布频率存在差异，即 PSDSD 和 PSDD 是两个具有不同症状群的抑郁亚型。

结论：本研究提出了新的 PSD 分类和诊断标准，这有利于 PSD 的早期识别和及时干预，从而使患者获得最佳治疗结局。

关键词：卒中后抑郁；分类；诊断标准

1　Introduction

　　Poststroke depression (PSD) is a common complication and is associated with increased physical disability, poor functional outcome and increased mortality. [1,2] It is very important to establish early recognition and rational diagnosis for this disease. However, studies on PSD have primarily focused on exploring its prevalence, pathogenic factors as well as treatment. [3-7] Only a few researchers have pursued the psychopathology and diagnosis of depression after stroke. [8,9] Like other psychiatric disorders, the diagnostic nosology was compelled to focus on clinical manifestations, duration and function disrupted due to ambiguous etiology. However, there are no accurate diagnostic and classified criteria in the following three diagnosis systems: the *Diagnostic and Statistical Manual of Mental Disorder*-Fifth Edition (DSM-5), the International Classification of Disease, Tenth Edition, and Chinese Classification of Mental Disorders, Third Version. It was also just described as "depressive disorder due to another medical condition" in the DSM-5 published in May 2013 (293.83). Regarding classification, some researchers put forward two forms of PSD, which are major and minor depression. The major depression is defined as MDD, while the minor depression is less well defined and usually diagnosed by dysthymic disorder. [10]

　　Previous results reported that the prevalence of PSD is $5\% \sim 67\%$ among all types of stroke patients. [11] This variation is influenced by the diagnostic criteria, evaluation instruments, different time intervals after the stroke, varied study populations, as well as the environment (hospital or community). [12,13] Among them, the nonstandard diagnostic criteria applied remain the main reasons for this broad range. The majority of previous studies used the contemporary diagnostic criteria of DSM-Ⅲ/Ⅳ and the structured clinical interviews,[14] while other studies used assessment scale as diagnostic criteria, which might be inappropriate.[15,16]

However, questions remain whether the same diagnostic criteria used in primary major depressive patients should be used in stroke survivors. First of all, the DSM-5 requires more than five depressive symptoms, with at least one of the symptoms being either:1) depressed mood or; 2) loss of interest or pleasure. Many depressed stroke patients will be rejected by using such strict demands. In the second place, some symptoms of diagnosing depression may occur in physically ill patients without depression[17] or some patients deny symptoms of depression due to anosognosia, cognitive dysfunction, neglect and pathological emotionalism.[18] Third, DSM-5 claims 2-week course of the depressive symptoms to diagnose major depressive disorder (MDD). It may miss the best observation period because average days of hospitalization were seven to ten in the Department of Neurology. For these reasons, some researchers debated that there is overdiagnosis or misdiagnosis using DSM as criteria to diagnose depression in stroke patients.[8,19] Therefore, we assume that the generalized PSD should include PSD symptoms (PSDS) and PSD disorder (PSDD) with different depressive characters, diagnostic criteria and treatment strategy. PSDS is the transition between normal and earliest manifestations of MDD, which describes the depressive state of individuals who do not fulfill MDD of the DSM-5 criteria. We further propose the ZhongDa diagnostic criteria-first edition (ZD-1) of PSDS based on the assessment scale (detailed in the "Methods" section).[20] Then, the individuals diagnosed with PSDS initiate antidepressant therapy to avoid the depressive progression and deterioration, while PSDD is considered as MDD after stroke.

The experience accumulated in the past few decades supports the notion that PSD is by no means a synonym of primary depression. Considering the insidious and progressive nature of mood disorders, we can put forward a new classification for PSD. The aim of the present study was to discuss the conceptual and practical aspects of diagnosis, assessment strategies and short-and long-term prognosis associated with different types of PSD.

2 Methods

2.1 Samples

Stroke inpatients were recruited from March 2015 to October 2015 in the Jiangsu province. All subjects provided written informed consent to participate in this study. The study was approved by the Medical Ethics Committee for Clinical Research of ZhongDa Hospital affiliated to Southeast University. A total of 166 patients who fulfilled the following criteria were recruited: 1) participants with ischemic stroke and intracerebral hemorrhage determined by computed tomography (CT) or magnetic resonance imaging (MRI); 2) participants evaluated with patient health questionnaire-9 (PHQ-9), PSD scale (PSD-S), mini-mental state examination (MMSE), National Institutes of Health Stroke Scale (NIHSS), modified Rankin scale (mRS), Barthel index (BI); 3) participants who were antidepressant-naïve; 4) participants free of depressive episode before stroke and other major psychiatric disorders, including schizophrenia, bipolar disorder, substance abuse (caffeine, nicotine and alcohol), neurodegenerative illness, severe physical illnesses and other medical illnesses; 5) participants free of vision, hearing and memory disorders and other symptoms that hindered assessment.

2.2 Classification and diagnosis of PSD

We put forward that the general PSD should include PSDS and PSDD according to each diagnostic criteria. The ZD-1 was established for PSDS considering the following problems. First, the symptoms of PSDS might be different from MDD, so we revised the symptoms in the diagnostic criteria for MDD in DSM-5 based on the suggestions of 65 Chinese chief doctors, keeping five general symptoms (easy to cry, insomnia, easy fatigability, feeling of decreased capability and suicidal ideation) and adding three specific symptoms (decreased speech, feeling of difficult to recover, more irritable than usual). Second, considering the incipient depression of PSD and the short hospitalization period of acute stroke patients, the course was adjusted to 1 week for early recognition of PSDS. Finally, we establish the diagnostic criteria of PSDS (Table 1) on the basis of the diagnostic framework for psychiatric disease. The differences between DSM-5 and ZD-1 are listed in Table 2. All participants were carefully analyzed and diagnosed as having PSDS and PSDD according to ZD-1 and DSM-5 criteria[21] by two trained participant neuropsychiatrists.

Table 1   Diagnostic criteria of ZhongDa (first edition) for PSDS

A. Three (or more) of the following symptoms have been present during the same 1-week period and represent a change from previous functioning.
   1. Decreased speech (eg, do not want to speak) most of the day, daily or most of the week.
   2. Fatigue or loss of energy daily or most of the week.
   3. Depressed mood persisting through the day, daily or most of the week, as indicated by either self-report or observation made by others (eg, feels sad, easy to cry).
   4. insomnia, wake up early or hypersomnia daily or most of the week.
   5. Feelings of decreased capability, worthlessness most of the day, daily or most of the week.
   6. Recurrent thoughts of death (not just fear of dying), recurrent suicidal ideation without a specific plan or a suicide attempt or a specific plan for committing suicide.
   7. Feeling of hopelessness or despair (especially feeling hard to recover from the disease) most of the day, daily or most of the week.
   8. More irritable than usual daily or most of the week.
B. The symptoms cause clinically significant distress or impairment in social interaction, occupation or other important areas of functioning.
C. The occurrence, development and duration of these symptoms are closely related to cerebrovascular disease.

D.	The occurrence of the major depressive episode could not be better explained by adjustment disorder with depressed mood, schizoaffective disorder, schizophrenia, schizophreniform disorder, delusional disorder, or other specified and unspecified schizophrenia spectrum and other psychotic disorders.
D.	No manic or a hypomanic episode is reported.

Abbreviation: PSDS, poststroke depression symptoms.

Table 2　Comparison of the DSM-5 and ZD-1 criteria

Items	DSM-5	ZD-1
Depressive symptoms		
Total depressive symptoms	9	8
Fulfilled depressive symptoms	5	3
Essential depressive symptoms	One of the symptoms is either 1) depressed mood or 2) loss of interest or pleasure	No
Duration	2 weeks	1 week

Abbreviations: DSM-5, Diagnostic and Statistical Manual of Mental Disorder-Fifth Edition; ZD-1, ZhongDa diagnostic criteria-first edition.

2.3　Statistical analysis

Data were described as mean and standard deviation (SD) for continuous variables, while classification variables were represented by number and percentage. The Statistical Package for the Social Sciences (SPSS) software version 20.0 (IBM Corp. Armonk, NY, USA) was used.

3　Results

3.1　Demographic and neuropsychological results

The majority of strokes (155, 93.98%) were classified as ischemic, with only 10 hemorrhagic strokes (6.02%). Sociodemographic and clinical variables of total participants are listed in Table 3. A total of 102 males and 64 females were included in the study, with a mean age of 64.37 (SD=10.85) and mean education level of 8. 49 (SD=4. 56). The mean scores of PSD-S and PHQ-9 were 6. 79 (SD=5. 61) and 6. 60 (SD=6. 07), respectively.

Table 3 Demographic and neuropsychological data of all participants

Item	PSDD(n=24)	PSDS(n=80)	Total(n=166)
Age (years)	64. 50±11. 26	64. 51±11. 96	64. 37±10. 85
Gender (male/female)	12/12	44/36	102/64
Education level (years)	8. 58±6. 93	8. 48±5. 25	8. 49±4. 56
PSD-S	15. 50±2. 81	10. 81±4. 69	6. 79±5. 61
PHQ-9	16. 38±3. 62	10. 73±5. 72	6. 60±6. 07
Stroke type (ischemic/hemorrhagic)	23/1	73/7	156/10
Neurological functional assessment			
NIHSS	3. 88±2. 31	3. 74±2. 87	2. 76±2. 73
mRS	2. 46±1. 18	2. 43±1. 25	1. 81±1. 28
BI	77. 29±21. 47	75. 00±23. 41	82. 95±22. 11
Vascular risk factors, n (%)			
Cardiovascular disease	20(83. 33)	62(77. 50)	126(75. 90)
Metabolic diseases	8(33. 33)	28(35. 00)	68(40. 96)
Active smokers	9(37. 50)	35(43. 75)	84(50. 60)
Alcohol consumption	7(29. 17)	19(23. 75)	47(28. 31)
Family history for stroke	0(0)	10(12. 50)	24(14. 46)

Note: Data reported as mean±SD and ratio.
Abbreviations: PSD-S, poststroke depression scale; PSDD, poststroke depression disorder; PSDS, poststroke depression symptoms; PHQ-9, patient health questionnaire-9; NIHSS, National Institutes of Health Stroke Scale; mRS, modified Rankin Scale; BI, Barthel index; SD, standard deviation.

The participants had mild or moderate stroke; the mean score of NIHSS was 2.76 (SD=2.73). The mean scores of mRS and BI reflecting neurological functions were 1.81 (SD=1.28) and 82.95 (SD=22.11), respectively. Twenty-four (14.46%) stroke patients had a family history of stroke.

Of all participants, 126 (75.90%) had cardiovascular disease and 68 (40.96%) had metabolic disease. A total of 84 (50.60%) stroke patients were active smokers, and 47 (28.31%) participants had the habit of alcohol consumption.

3.2 Subtypes of PSD diagnosed by different diagnostic criteria

A total of 80 (48.19%) patients were diagnosed with PSDS according to ZD-1 including 24 PSDD and 56 patients who did not meet the diagnostic criteria by DSM-5 (Table 4). The patients diagnosed with PSDS should satisfy the ZD-1 diagnostic criteria first. The depressive severity of PSDS was lower than PSDD by the PHQ-9 (10.81±4.69 vs 15.50±2.81) and PSD-S (10.73±5.72 vs 16.38±3.62).

Table 4　Subtypes of PSD patients according to different diagnostic criteria

Subtypes of PSD	PSDD (DSM-5 diagnostic criteria)		Total
	Yes	No	
PSDS (ZD-1 diagnostic criteria)			
Yes	24	56	80
No	0	86	86
Total	24	142	166

Abbreviations: PSD, poststroke depression; PSDD, poststroke depression disorder; DSM-5, *Diagnostic and Statistical Manual of Mental Disorder* – Fifth edition; PSDS, poststroke depression symptoms; ZD-1, ZhongDa diagnostic criteria – first edition.

The symptoms in the DSM-5 (nine items) and ZD-1 (eight items) have 17 items together containing three same symptoms (insomnia, waking up too early; fatigue or loss of energy; suicidal ideation). The frequency of the remaining 14 symptoms in three groups is reported in Table 5. The depressive symptoms of first five-sevenths distribution frequency were located in ZD-1 (Decreased speech, Feeling of decreased capability, Feeling of difficult to recover, Fatigue or loss of energy and Insomnia or hypersomnia), while only two symptoms in DSM-5 ranked in first seven items (Depressed mood and Diminished interest or pleasure).

Table 5 Symptom profile of PSD and total patients

Item	PSDD ($n=24$)	PSDS ($n=80$)	Total ($n=166$)
Decreased speech (item 1), $n(\%)$	21(87.50)	53(66.25)	73(43.98)
Easy to cry (item 2), $n(\%)$	17(70.83)	36(45.00)	43(25.90)
Feeling of decreased capability (item 3), $n(\%)$	20(83.33)	67(83.75)	101(60.84)
Feeling of difficult to recover (item 4), $n(\%)$	22(91.67)	56(70.00)	65(39.16)
More irritable than usual (item 5), $n(\%)$	16(66.67)	37(46.25)	46(27.71)
Fatigue or loss of energy (item 6), $n(\%)$	22(91.67)	68(85.00)	106(63.86)
Insomnia or hypersomnia (item 7), $n(\%)$	22(91.67)	46(57.50)	61(36.75)
Recurrent thoughts of death (item 8), $n(\%)$	8(33.33)	12(15.00)	14(8.43)
Depressed mood (item 9), $n(\%)$	24(100.00)	58(72.50)	76(45.78)
Diminished interest or pleasure (item 10), $n(\%)$	23(95.83)	45(56.25)	61(36.75)
Significant weight loss when not dieting or weight gain (item 11), $n(\%)$	17(70.83)	36(45.00)	40(24.10)
Psychomotor agitation or retardation (item 12), $n(\%)$	13(54.17)	38(47.50)	50(30.12)
Feelings of worthlessness or excessive or inappropriate guilt (item 13), $n(\%)$	16(66.67)	39(48.75)	47(28.31)
Diminished ability to think or concentrate, or indecisiveness (item 14), $n(\%)$	18(75.00)	35(43.75)	52(31.33)

Abbreviations: PSD, poststroke depression; PSDD, poststroke depression disorder; PSDS, poststroke depression symptoms.

From Table 6, we can find that if we use five symptoms and 2 weeks of the ZD-1 as diagnostic criteria, 27 patients were incorporated in PSDD, which is similar to DSM-5. However, when we adopt three symptoms and 1 week as diagnostic criteria, 80 depression patients fulfilled these criteria. The detection rate of depressive patients increased from 16.27% to 48.19%.

Table 6　Patients fulfilled different depressive symptoms and duration of the ZD-1 diagnostic criteria

Duration	ZD-1 diagnostic criteria		
	More than five symptoms	More than four symptoms	More than three symptoms
More than 14 days	27	31	36
7—13 days	14	28	44
0—6 days	3	10	19
Total	44	69	99

Abbreviation: ZD-1, ZhongDa diagnostic criteria – first edition.

4　Discussion

The present study had two major findings. 1) We proposed the clear classification of PSD including PSDS and PSDD (Figure 1). PSDS described the depressive state of individuals who report emotional problems but do not reach the diagnostic criteria for MDD, which should preferably be defined and corroborated. PSDD was considered as the patients who fulfilled the criterion of major depression after stroke. 2) We highlighted the importance of formal diagnostic criteria for the purpose of identifying stroke patients who have signs of depression. The clear category provided the basis for subsequent diagnosis and treatment.

Although PSDD was widely accepted and defined in MDD criteria of DSM-Ⅳ,[22] this viewpoint was argued by some investigators.[23,24] In order to avoid neglecting the depressive stroke survivors down to the diagnostic criteria of MDD, Robinson et al[25] suggested dividing depression into major and minor types according to different criteria in the 1980s. However, it will result in problems with the diagnostic criteria of dysthymia for mild PSD, such that it not only lost sight of the essential issue with distinct symptoms of these two depression types but also missed the best opportunity of clinical intervention for a standard long course. Therefore, we suggested that PSD should consist of PSDS and PSDD with different depressive characters, diagnostic criteria and treatment strategy. PSDS is the incipient depression or the earlier stages of PSD, which can progress to PSDD, maintain its original condition or alleviate by itself. At this point, it is particularly important for timely effective intervention for preventing the situation from worsening.

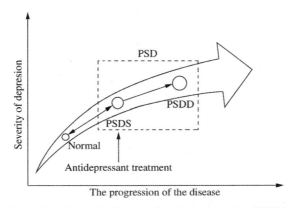

Figure 1   schematic diagram for the progression of PSD.

Notes: The generalized PSD should include PSDS and PSDD with different depressive characters and diagnostic criteria. PSDS is the transition between normal and PSDD, which represents the incipient depression or the earlier stages of PSD. it can progress to PSDD, maintain its original condition or alleviate by itself. The individuals diagnosed with PSDS initiate antidepressant therapy to avoid the depressive progression and deterioration, whereas PSDD is considered as MDD after stroke.

Abbreviations: PSD, poststroke depression; PSDS, poststroke depression symptoms; PSDD, poststroke depression disorder; MDD, major depressive disorder.

There are several important issues that need to be addressed in evaluating diagnostic criteria. 1) must be ascertained if these proposed modified diagnostic criteria are valid before adopting this new standard. A total of 27 patients were diagnosed with PSDD if we use five depressive symptoms and 2 weeks of ZD-1 as criteria, which is similar to the existing DSM-IV criteria. This indirectly evidenced that the standards of ZD-1 were equivalent to DSM-5.

2) These criteria are based on the specific symptom or a group of phenomenological characteristics that differentiate between patients with and without the disease. Our results of five-sevenths top ranking symptoms distributing in ZD-1 manifested that the clusters of symptoms to predict PSDS are rational. Previous literature has demonstrated that crying and overt sadness are more reliable indicators of depression than apathy in the stroke unit. [26] Our investigation also proved this point by prior knowledge of chief clinicians when we established the assessment scale. In spite of the fact that the two symptoms, loss of energy and feeling of difficult to recover, were also the most common characteristics in depressed and total patients, the percentages in depression group were larger than those of total participants. Similar changes were found in another study that PSD individuals have a high frequency of vegetative symptoms such as loss of energy and early awakening. [27,28] Combined with this finding and previous knowledge, the ZD-1 diagnostic criteria demarcating from primary depression was good for PSDS patients. Notwithstanding, it will be better if we modulate the item of easy to cry to depressed mood covering extensive scope.

3) The course of PSDS was defined as 1 week for early recognition to facilitate the hospitalization period of acute stroke patients considering the following two reasons. On the one hand, the validity of diagnostic catego-

ries is ultimately on account of sharing similarities in etiology of all patients. The etiology of PSD is relatively specific with stroke, so we could rather easily establish the truly rational diagnosis. On the other hand, the previous study demonstrated that the prevalence of depression appeared stable during the immediate week and 3 months following the stroke, although depressive symptom profiles are likely to be different. [29] We also displayed that 19 depressed stroke patients with three symptoms did not last 7 days. Further studies of the ambulatory of depression and the duration of PSDS<7 days are needed.

4) The diagnostic categories are the prerequisite of the treatment response and remission. Standard antidepressant treatment should be initiated once a diagnosis of PSDD was confirmed. [30] But today there is not enough evidence to recommend a preventive therapy for depression in any stroke patient though it shows improvement trends. [31,32] Presentation of PSDS provides clear treatment indications for those patients with depressive symptoms. Early recognition and standard diagnosis of PSD are the preconditions of timely treatment and largest neurological and social functional recovery. [33,34]

Our exploratory research has several limitations. 1) Our sample was relatively small, the large population and classificatory research would be conducted in the further study. 2) The present study was a cross-sectional study; dynamic change in depression may be better presented by a follow-up study. 3) Patients included in our study were those with mild or moderate stroke, which might make a circumscribed applicability.

5 Conclusion

The present study put the new opinion that PSD could be divided into two types, PSDS and PSDD. PSDS is the transition between normal and PSDD, which is diagnosed by the new established ZD-1 criteria, whereas the diagnosis of PSDD is most appropriately based on DSM-5 criteria for depression due to stroke with the major depressive-like episode. Awareness of depression in stroke survivors with different subtypes represents a deep comprehension of this disease, and it is essential for early recognition, long-term management and implementation of effective interventions.

6 Acknowledgments

This work was supported by Jiangsu Provincial Special Program of Medical Science (BL2012025, Yonggui Yuan), The foundation for excellent doctorial dissertations of Southeast University (YBJJ1539), the Fundamental Research Funds for the Central Universities and the Ordinary University Graduate Student Scientific Research Innovation Project of Jiangsu province (KYZZ15_0064). We thank all individuals who participated in this study.

7 Disclosure

The authors report no conflicts of interest in this work.

References

[1] Schmid AA, Kroenke K, Hendrie HC, Bakas T, Sutherland JM, Williams LS. Poststroke depression and treatment effects on functional outcomes. Neurology, 2011,76(11):1000 – 1005.

[2] Pompili M, Venturini P, Campi S, et al. Do stroke patients have an increased risk of developing suicidal ideation or dying by suicide? An overview of the current literature. CNS Neurosci Ther. 2012,18(9):711 – 721.

[3] Altieri M, Maestrini I, Mercurio A, et al. Depression after minor stroke: preva-

lence and predictors. Eur J Neurol. 2012,19(3):517 - 521.

[4] Srivastava ATA, Gupta A, Murali T. Post-stroke depression: prevalence and relationship with disability in chronic stroke survivors. Ann Indian Acad Neurol. 2010, 13(2):123 - 127.

[5] Zhang T, Wang C, Liu L, et al. A prospective cohort study of the incidence and determinants of post-stroke depression among the mainland Chinese patients. Neurol Res. 2010,32(4):347 - 352.

[6] Zhang N, Wang CX, Wang AX, et al. Time course of depression and one-year prognosis of patients with stroke in mainland China. CNS Neurosci Ther. 2012,18 (6):475 - 481.

[7] Narushima K, Kosier JT, Robinson RG. Preventing poststroke depression: a 12-week double-blind randomized treatment trial and 21-month follow-up. J Nerv Ment Dis. 2002,190(5):296 - 303.

[8] Fedoroff JP, Starkstein SE, Parikh RM, Price TR, Robinson RG. Are depressive symptoms nonspecific in patients with acute stroke? Am J Psychiatry. 1991,148 (9):1172 - 1176.

[9] Turner A, Hambridge J, White J, et al. Depression screening in stroke: a comparison of alternative measures with the structured diagnostic interview for the diagnostic and statistical manual of mental disorders, fourth edition (major depressive episode) as criterion standard. Stroke. 2012,43(4):1000 - 1005.

[10] Morris PL, Shields RB, Hopwood MJ, Robinson RG, Raphael B. Are there two depressive syndromes after stroke? J Nerv Ment Dis. 1994,182(4):230 - 234.

[11] Ferro JM, Caeiro L, Santos C. Poststroke emotional and behavior impairment: a narrative review. Cerebrovasc Dis. 2009,27:197 - 203.

[12] Lees R, Stott DJ, Quinn TJ, Broomfield NM. Feasibility and diagnostic accuracy of early mood screening to diagnose persisting clinical depression/anxiety disorder after stroke. Cerebrovasc Dis. 2014,37(5): 323 - 329.

[13] Astrom M, Adolfsson R, Asplund K. Major depression in stroke patients. A 3-year longitudinal study. Stroke. 1993,24(7):976 - 982.

[14] Robinson RG, Jorge RE. Post-stroke depression: a review. Am J Psychiatry.

2016,173(3):221 - 231.

[15] Desmond DW, Remien RH, Moroney JT, Stern Y, Sano M, Williams JB. Ischemic stroke and depression. J Int Neuropsychol Soc. 2003,9(3):429 - 439.

[16] Ayerbe L, Ayis S, Rudd AG, Heuschmann PU, Wolfe CD. Natural history, predictors, and associations of depression 5 years after stroke: the South London Stroke Register. Stroke. 2011,42(7):1907 - 1911.

[17] Rodin G, Voshart K. Depression in the medically ill: an overview. Am J Psychiatry. 1986,143(6):696 - 705.

[18] House A, Dennis M, Mogridge L, Warlow C, Hawton K, Jones L. Mood disorders in the year after first stroke. Br J Psychiatry. 1991,158: 83 - 92.

[19] Cumming TB, Churilov L, Skoog I, Blomstrand C, Linden T. Little evidence for different phenomenology in poststroke depression. Acta Psychiatr Scand. 2010, 121(6):424 - 430.

[20] Yue Y, Liu R, Lu J, et al. Reliability and validity of a new post-stroke depression scale in Chinese population. J Affect Disord. 2015,174: 317 - 323.

[21] American Psychiatric Association. Diagnostic and Statistical Manual of Mental Disorders-DSM-5. Washington, DC: American Psychiatric Press, Inc. 2013.

[22] Spalletta G, Robinson RG. How should depression be diagnosed in patients with stroke? Acta Psychiatr Scand. 2010,121(6):401 - 403.

[23] da Rocha e Silva CE, Alves Brasil MA, Matos do Nascimento E, de Braganca Pereira B, Andre C. Is poststroke depression a major depression? Cerebrovasc Dis. 2013,35(4):385 - 391.

[24] Maj M. When does depression become a mental disorder? Br J Psychiatry. 2011, 199(2):85 - 86.

[25] Robinson RG, Bolduc PL, Price TR. Two-year longitudinal study of poststroke mood disorders: diagnosis and outcome at one and two years. Stroke. 1987, 18 (5):837 - 843.

[26] Carota A, Berney A, Aybek S, et al. A prospective study of predictors of poststroke depression. Neurology. 2005,64(3):428 - 433.

[27] Tateno A, Kimura M, Robinson RG. Phenomenological characteristics of posts-

troke depression: early-versus late-onset. Am J Geriatr Psychiatry. 2002,10(5):
575 – 582.

[28] Paradiso S, Ohkubo T, Robinson RG. Vegetative and psychological symptoms associated with depressed mood over the first two years after stroke. Int J Psychiatry Med. 1997,27(2):137 – 157.

[29] Sibon I, Lassalle-Lagadec S, Renou P, Swendsen J. Evolution of depression symptoms following stroke: a prospective study using computerized ambulatory monitoring. Cerebrovasc Dis. 2012,33(3):280 – 285.

[30] Robinson RG. Poststroke depression: prevalence, diagnosis, treatment, and disease progression. Biol Psychiatry. 2003,54(3):376 – 387.

[31] Gabaldon L, Fuentes B, Frank-Garcia A, Diez-Tejedor E. Poststroke depression: importance of its detection and treatment. Cerebrovasc Dis. 2007,24(suppl 1):181 – 188.

[32] Chen Y, Patel NC, Guo JJ, Zhan S. Antidepressant prophylaxis for poststroke depression: a meta-analysis. Int Clin Psychopharmacol. 2007,22(3):159 – 166.

[33] Flaster M, Sharma A, Rao M. Poststroke depression: a review emphasizing the role of prophylactic treatment and synergy with treatment for motor recovery. Top Stroke Rehabil. 2013,20(2):139 – 150.

[34] Van de Meent H, Geurts AC, Van Limbeek J. Pharmacologic treatment of poststroke depression: a systematic review of the literature. Top Stroke Rehabil. 2003, 10(1):79 – 92.

[作者及发表刊物:

Yingying Yue, Rui Liu, Yin Cao, Yanfeng Wu, shining Zhang, Huajie Li, Jijun Zhu, Wenhao Jiang, Aiqin Wu, Yonggui Yuan. New opinion on the subtypes of poststroke depression in Chinese stroke survivors[J]. Neuropsychiatr Dis Treat. 2017,13:707 – 713.]

中国卒中后抑郁障碍规范化诊疗指南

1　概述

卒中后抑郁障碍（post-stroke depression，PSD）是在卒中发生后出现的以抑郁症状群为主要临床特征的心境障碍，是卒中的常见并发症之一，自20世纪80年代以来引起了越来越多的临床医师及研究者的重视。

PSD 和原发性抑郁症（major depressive disorder，MDD）的临床表现相似，但一些症状的发生频率有一定差别：MDD 患者中快感缺失、悲观和自杀想法及严重的注意力不集中等症状十分常见；而 PSD 患者中情绪波动、迟缓、激越、情感淡漠则较为多见[1, 2]。需要注意的是，迟缓、淡漠等症状本身也可能是卒中后神经功能缺损的表现，易与抑郁相混淆。自罪、自杀观念及行为、体重减轻及早醒等症状对 PSD 诊断缺乏特异性[3]。PSD 会降低卒中患者的运动功能及生活质量[4]，同时明显提高卒中幸存者自杀的风险[5]。对 PSD 患者早期使用抗抑郁治疗能够促进其运动及认知功能的恢复，并进一步提高卒中后存活年数至十年[6]。因此，寻找并识别特异于 PSD 的抑郁症状是十分重要而艰巨的任务。

2014 年一篇 meta 分析示卒中后 5 年内 PSD 的发生率约为 31%[7]，然而一篇系统综述报道，在所有类型的卒中患者中，PSD 的发病率介于 5% 至 67%[8]。根据国内一例相关研究，PSD 的发病率为 45.79%，其中 34.21% 为早发型 PSD，11.58% 为晚发型 PSD（发生在卒中 2 周后）[9]。在大部分研究中，早发型 PSD 被定义为发生在卒中后 2 周内的 PSD，而晚发型 PSD 则发生在卒中 2 周后[9-11]。然而在国内另一项研究中，PSD 的发病率为 25%—79%[12]。多个因素导致了这些不一致的研究结果：首先，不同的研究采用的 PSD 诊断标准不一致，采用评估量表作为诊断标准的研究 PSD 发病率高于采用精神障碍诊断标准的研究[13,14]；其次，对卒中患者的评估阶段不同导致 PSD 的发生率存在差异[15-17]，多数 PSD 都发生在卒中的急性期，而在随访过程中,新发 PSD 的数量则会下降[10];再次,评估人群和评估地点的不同也会导致发病率存在差异,研究发现神经科和康复中心的患者 PSD 发病率明显高于社区医院患者[18];最后,卒中导致的失语、失认、认知功能受损等也会增加 PSD 的识别和诊断的复杂性,造成一定程度的漏诊和误诊。

广义的 PSD 包括卒中后抑郁症状(post stroke depressive symptoms,PSDS)和卒中后抑郁症(post stroke depressive disorder,PSDD),前者强调抑郁和卒中平行发展,关系密切,抑郁可以是卒中直接脑损伤所致,或是卒中后的急性心理社会反应;后者则更可能是卒中诱发的(内源性)抑郁症,常于卒中半年后发生,可以由卒中或者卒中后遗症诱发。

PSDS 持续时间较短,平均为 12 周,而 PSDD 的平均病程可持续 39 周[19]。卒中后 6 个月内新发的 PSD 患者在 3~6 个月内缓解率超过 50%,但有相当一部分患者会在 1 年内复发[16]。PSD 会影响卒中后的日常活动功能和认知功能的恢复,且合并认知功能损害者的神经功能恢复更差[20-22]。2016 年国内一项调查发现抑郁和卒中后 5 年残疾率相关[23]。PSD 患者在卒中的急性期及中晚期的自杀观念发生率分别为 6.6% 和 11.3%[24]。近来一项全国性研究发现 PSD 可能是卒中所致死亡的独立危险因素[25]。

全球疾病负担(2013)研究显示[26]:2013 年全球有 1.03 亿新发卒中患者(67% 为缺血性),其中有 650 万人死于脑卒中(51% 源于缺血性脑卒中),相关伤残调整寿命年(disability-adjusted life years,DALYs)为 1130 万(58% 源于缺血性脑卒中)。2010 年卒中在我国造成 170 万人死亡,相关 DALYs 为 210 万[27]。2005 年我国脑卒中的直接经济负担为 198.87 亿元,占国家医疗总费用的 3.79%,占国家卫生总费用的 3.02%[28]。目前,尚无直接对 PSD 疾病负担进行调查的研究[29],但考虑到 PSD 较高的发生率、死亡率以及其对卒中功能恢复的显著影响,可以推测抑郁对卒中后疾病负担的影响较大。

虽然 PSD 对卒中幸存者和医疗工作人员都是一项严重的问题,但是目前国内仍然没有形成针对 PSD 临床管理的标准化指南。在国内临床工作中,PSD 患者常常被误诊或漏诊,也因此无法获得及时而有效的治疗。即使现有的抗抑郁治疗能够改善抑郁症状,最优的药物选择及治疗时程依然难以确定[30]。

2　PSD 危险因素

PSD 的发生受年龄[31]、性别[32]、种族与文化背景[33]及受教育程度[34]等多种因素影响,然而不同研究的结果存在不一致,目前尚无确切结论。

卒中后的躯体功能障碍,以及由此带来的工作及生活能力丧失、社会或家庭地位的改变是 PSD 发生的主要社会心理应激因素[35]。应激生活事件[13]、缺乏社会支持[36]、较低的家庭经济收入[37]、病前神经质人格[38]、A 型行为[39]可增加 PSD 发病风险。

家族史是 PSD 发生的主要危险因素之一[17]。分子遗传学研究表明与 PSD 有关的基因包括:5-羟色胺(5-serotonin transporter,5-HT)转运体[40]、5-HT 1A[41]与 2A[42]受体、脑源性神经营养因子(brain-derived neurotrophic factor,BDNF)[43]、N5,N10-亚甲基四氢叶酸还原酶(N5,N10 methylenetetrahydrorolate reductase,MTHFR)[44]、儿茶酚氧位甲基转移酶(catechol-O-methyltransferase,COMT)[45]、白介素 10(interleukin-10,IL-10)与 IL-4[46]及 cAMP 反应元件结合蛋白(cAMP response element binding protein,CREB)[47]等相关基因。其中研究较多的是 5-HT 转运体及 5-HT 受体相关基因,基因-基因、基因-环境交互作用也参与 PSD 的发病[43]。此外,微小 RNA 在 PSD 发生及抗抑郁治疗过程中也扮演关键角色[48]。

神经递质的改变是当前 PSD 研究的热门领域,脑卒中后急性期 PSD 患者脑脊液中去甲肾上腺素、5-HT 以及 5-HT 的代谢产物 5-羟基吲哚乙酸(5-hydroxyindole acetic acid,5-HIAA)的含量明显下降[49,50];氢质子磁共振波谱研究发现 PSD 患者存在前额叶谷氨酸代谢的异常[51]。

炎症反应可能参与 PSD 发病,卒中后致炎性细胞因子(如 IL-1、IL-6、IL-18、TNF-α 等)增多[52],血清 C 反应蛋白水平可作为 PSD 发生及严重程度的重要预测因子[53]。

神经内分泌研究提示，PSD 患者存在下丘脑-垂体-肾上腺轴、下丘脑-垂体-甲状腺轴及下丘脑-垂体-性腺轴异常[54, 55]。此外，PSD 的发生与血清 BDNF 水平降低[56]、铁蛋白[57]和新蝶呤水平升高[58]有关。

神经解剖异常在 PSD 的发病中起重要作用，PSD 的发生可能与调节情绪的额颞叶-基底节-腹侧脑干环路受损及相关的神经化学递质异常有关[59]。目前该领域研究主要围绕脑卒中损伤病灶和脑白质疏松两方面。脑卒中损伤病灶与 PSD 的关系至今仍是极富争议的研究领域，不同研究结果相互矛盾。可能的解释是，不同临床特征 PSD 所对应的脑卒中损伤部位并不一致，情感性抑郁的严重性与左额叶损伤相关，而淡漠性抑郁的严重性则与双侧基底节损伤相关[60]。损伤部位与额极的距离也和 PSD 的频率和严重程度相关，研究发现，损伤部位离额极越近，抑郁就越严重[61]。且以疾病的不同时期进行亚组分析的结果示急性期（卒中后 1 个月内）左半球卒中患者易罹患 PSD，而亚急性期（卒中后 1～6 个月）右半球卒中的患者易罹患 PSD[62]。此外，脑白质疏松可能在梗死灶较小的 PSD 发生中起较为重要的作用，而梗死灶较大患者中的病灶本身作用更大[63]。

3 PSD 临床评估

PSD 的早期识别、预防和治疗对脑卒中患者的康复和预后非常重要。PSD 有多重危险因素，其完整评估应包括一般情况、卒中功能和抑郁症状等方面。

3.1 一般情况评估

3.1.1 现病史

脑卒中急性期抑郁症状的筛查十分重要，应全面评估抑郁的发生时间、特点、严重程度、伴随的其他精神与躯体症状。考虑到 PSD 与卒中关系密切，还应该详细评估卒中的病变性质、部位、大小、严重程度及卒中后患者的功能状态。

3.1.2 既往史

既往脑卒中病史、抑郁症和其他精神疾病病史是预测 PSD 的重要因素，应详细评估是否存在这些疾病以及其相应的治疗情况;此外,还应该了解患者的血管危险因素,如高血压、心绞痛是 PSD 发病的独立预测因素[64,65]。

3.1.3　个人史及家族史

评估应重点关注性别、年龄、生活事件、家庭经济收入、独居、社会支持、神经质人格[66-68]等和 PSD 发病密切相关的因素。另外还应仔细询问卒中患者是否有抑郁症家族史。

3.2　卒中功能评定

卒中严重的后果之一是导致肢体功能障碍,常用评定量表包括美国国立卫生院神经功能缺损评分量表[69]、改良 Rankin 量表[70]及 Barthel 指数评定量表[71]。

3.3　抑郁症状评估

临床上用于抑郁症状评估的工具包括自评量表和他评量表两种。常用的自评量表包括宗氏抑郁自评量表(self-rating depression scale, SDS)[72]、贝克抑郁自评量表(Beck depression inventory, BDI)[73]、9 条目健康问卷(patient health questionnaire-9, PHQ-9)[74]、医院焦虑抑郁量表(hospital anxiety and depression scale, HADS)[75]及流调用抑郁自评量表(center for epidemiologic studies depression scale, CES-D)[76]。常用的他评量表包括汉密尔顿抑郁量表[77]和蒙哥马利-艾森博格抑郁评价量表(Montgomery-Asberg depression rating scale, MADRS)[78]。

上述量表均是为 MDD 评估而设计,考虑到 PSD 与 MDD 的症状差异,用于 PSD 的评估缺乏特异性。袁勇贵课题组在既往量表的基础上,制定卒中后抑郁障碍评估量表(post stroke depression scale, PSD-S),该量表为自评量表,有较好的同质性信度(Cronbach's $\alpha = 0.797$)和区分效度[79],6/24、15/24 分别为轻度、中重度 PSD,可以用于 PSD 的普遍筛查(见附录 2)。PHQ-9 是由 DSM-5 衍生的抑郁筛查工具,由抑郁症诊断的 9 条症状学标准构成,评估过去 2 周症状出现的频率。Williams 等[80]将 PHQ-9 在卒中人群进行抑郁筛查研究,结果显示以 4 分为截点,PHQ-9 的灵敏度为 91%,特异度为 89%。该量表简单易用,而且信效度好,亦被推荐用于抑郁症及 PSD 患者的筛查(见附录 2)。

4 PSD 诊断及鉴别诊断

目前国际上通用的精神疾病分类体系均未对 PSD 给出明确的诊断标准,部分相关研究使用 MDD 诊断标准,或仅依靠抑郁评估量表的评定结果作为诊断标准。2013 年出版的 DSM-5 则将这类患者归为"由于其他躯体疾病所致的抑郁障碍(293.83)",并将其分为伴抑郁特征(F06.31),伴类重型抑郁发作(F06.32)和伴混合特征(F06.34)[81]。

临床上 PSD 可分为 PSDS 和 PSDD,PSDS 是介于正常和 PSDD 的中间过渡状态,该状态既可以继续发展为 PSDD,也可以维持原状或自行缓解(图1)[82]。袁勇贵课题组首次提出 PSDS 的诊断标准(表 1),在卒中后一周时即可对患者进行诊断评估,而 PSDD 即卒中后的抑郁症,其诊断需首先满足 PSDS 的诊断标准,同时符合 DSM-5 中 MDD 诊断标准[79]。为了明确诊断,PSD 应与卒中后淡漠、卒中后焦虑、卒中后疲劳及卒中后精神障碍等相鉴别。

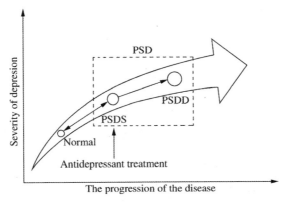

图 1 PSD 进展的示意图[82]

卒中后淡漠和 PSD 有很多相似之处,常易混淆,但可从以下几方面进行区分:精神症状学方面,情感淡漠与脱抑制状态、认知功能下降以及异常运动行为相关,而抑郁与焦虑、激动、易激惹等情绪相关[83];情感性质方面,情感淡漠患者呈现出一种漠不关心的状态,其心境为中性,一般不会有自杀念头[84],而抑郁患者呈明显的负性心境;面部表情方面,淡漠者常表情平淡,目光空洞,缺乏眼神交流,而抑郁者常有典型的愁苦伤心的面容,目光可以含有感情。

卒中后焦虑(post-stroke anxiety, PSA)常见于卒中慢性期,且随着病程延长,发病率逐渐上升[85],而 PSD 在急性期更常见;PSD 发病与卒中前是否患抑郁关系不大,更多受到卒中这一负性事件本身的影响,而 PSA 与病前焦虑关系密切[86];PSD 主要表现为持续的抑郁情绪,兴趣减少,可伴有心慌、紧张、担心等躯体性焦虑或精神性焦虑,但抑郁心境是 PSD 的核心症状,PSA 表现为发作性恐惧、紧张、担心、易激惹、坐立不安等焦虑症状。

卒中后疲劳(post stroke fatigue,PSF)是躯体或心理能量缺乏而影响自主活动的一种主观感受到的身体或心理的疲倦,具有异常性、过渡性、慢性的特点,与之前是否做过运动或活动无关[87]。脑卒中疲劳如果出现情绪差或 PSD 伴随有全身无力躯体症状或有精力减退等抑郁的典型症状,常常需要对二者加以鉴别。

卒中后精神障碍是卒中急性期、恢复期及后遗症期发生的多种精神症状,急性期易并发以抑郁最为常见,其他包括幻觉、妄想、异常兴奋的精神障碍,影响患者的康复和生活质量[88]。卒中后精神障碍一般进展缓慢,病程波动,可因卒中而急性加剧,也可因侧支循环代偿而好转,其临床表现多样,最终常发展为痴呆。

表 1　PSDS 诊断标准

A.	在同样的 1 周时期内,出现 3 个或以上的下列症状,表现出与先前功能相比不同的变化。

　　1. 几乎每天或每天的大部分时间都言语减少(不想说话);

　　2. 几乎每天都易疲乏或精力减退;

　　3. 几乎每天或每天的大部分时间都心境抑郁,主观描述及他人观察均可(例如感到悲伤,容易哭泣);

　　4. 几乎每天都失眠、早醒或睡眠过多;

　　5. 几乎每天或每天的大部分时间都感到自己能力下降;

　　6. 反复出现想死的念头或有自杀、自伤行为;

　　7. 几乎每天或每天的大部分时间都感觉自己好不了;

　　8. 几乎每天都比平常容易生气激动。

B.　这些症状引起临床意义的痛苦,或导致社交、职业或其他重要功能方面的损害。

C.　这些症状的发生、发展及病程与脑血管疾病密切相关。

D.　这种抑郁发作的出现不能更好地用适应障碍伴抑郁心境,分裂情感性障碍,精神分裂症,精神分裂症样障碍,妄想障碍,或其他特定的或未特定的精神分裂症谱系及其他精神病性障碍来解释。

E.　从无躁狂发作或轻躁狂发作。

5　PSD 的治疗

5.1　药物治疗

　　及时合理的抗抑郁治疗不仅有助于 PSD 患者抑郁症状恢复,对其神经功能康复也有积极影响,并能改善长期预后。PSD 的治疗应该以良好的医患关系为基础,建立包括患者及家属在内的治疗联盟,争取得到患者及家属主动配合,共同致力于患者的健康恢复。建议当患者满足 PSDS 诊断标准时,即可开始给予抗抑郁治疗,包括药物治疗、物理治疗、心理治疗等。

　　PSD 患者首选抗抑郁剂治疗[89]。根据 PSD 患者抑郁的症状选择相应的抗抑郁药物,了解可能存在的药物副反应,特别是对于老年人,要充分掌握所选药物与其他现服药物的相互作用及其对现患疾病的影响。考虑到抗抑郁药的某些副反应,患者的耐受性会有所下降[89]。因此临床医生应密切观察患者对治疗的反应,计划好定期的评估和保持警惕,时刻关注可能发生的药物副作用,与患者充分沟通增加其治疗依从性。另外,患者在治疗 PSD 过程中也存在躁狂发作的风险,一旦发现这种情况,应立刻减量或停用抗抑郁剂,并加用情感稳定剂。

在抗抑郁剂治疗方面,一项纳入 788 例 PSD 患者的多中心、随机、对照研究表明帕罗西汀治疗 8 周的显效率达 93.1%[90]。西酞普兰[91]、艾司西酞普兰[92]、舍曲林[93]、氟伏沙明[94]及米氮平[95]等抗抑郁药仅得到少数临床研究支持。纳入 11 项随机对照研究的 Meta 分析提示氟西汀对 PSD 有较好的疗效[96];而另一项纳入 32 项随机对照研究的 Meta 分析证实文拉法辛对 PSD 的疗效优于选择性 5-羟色胺再摄取抑制剂(selective serotonin re-uptake inhibitors,SSRIs)药物[98]。然而,这些研究样本量较小或并非 RCT 研究,故证据效力不足。

中医药也被应用于 PSD 的治疗。轻度抑郁可以单用中药治疗,中重度抑郁可以联合抗抑郁药治疗。目前有临床研究结果支持的、可用于 PSD 治疗的中药制剂包括乌灵胶囊及舒肝解郁胶囊[99, 100]。

但是,关于抗抑郁治疗的时效性目前存在争议。Fruehwald 等[101]在一项随访研究中发现,卒中后服用三个月氟西汀的 PSD 患者 18 个月时的情绪改善及功能恢复状况甚为明显,而早期服药时则与对照组无明显差异。一项针对中国人群的随机单盲临床研究发现,卒中患者早期服用 3 个月西酞普兰,其抗抑郁效果在卒中 6 个月后更显著[102]。这些研究结果提示,早期服药的效果可能为多种临床因素所掩盖,PSD 是否需要像抑郁症一样进行急性期、巩固期和维持期足疗程治疗,仍需进一步研究证实。加拿大 2015 年卒中最佳实践指南建议如果所选药物有效,应该继续治疗至少 6～12 个月[103]。针对 PSDS 而言,维持治疗时间可以适当缩短,一般在抑郁症状消失再继续治疗 2～3 个月。

5.2 物理治疗

重复经颅磁刺激(repetitive transcranial magnetic stimulation,rTMS)对难治性 PSD 患者的疗效及安全性均较好[104],建议卒中半年后进行 rTMS

治疗,对于 PSD 治疗的优化频率及刺激强度有待更多的临床证据证实。rTMS常见的副作用包括头痛、胃肠道反应、口干、震颤甚至癫痫发作[105]。电休克治疗(electroconvulsive therapy,ECT)可用于具有严重自杀念头、对药物不能耐受和难治性的非急性期 PSD 患者。但 ECT 常导致或加重认知功能障碍,且易出现 ECT 相关并发症,故不作为 PSD 的首选治疗[106]。早期开展积极的肢体康复治疗有利于 PSD 患者的长期预后。但是许多卒中幸存者,尤其是脑出血或者置入支架的患者,可能无法耐受 rTMS 或者 ECT,需要注意相关的副反应。

5.3 心理治疗

支持性心理治疗及认知行为治疗对 PSD 有效[107, 108]。社会支持包括家庭、朋友、同事等多探视陪伴病人,给以安慰、关心,鼓励病人积极配合治疗及进行康复锻炼。社会支持有利于患者重返社会,重建人与人之间的良好关系,可防止 PSD 的发生或减轻其程度。认知行为治疗(cognitive behavior therapy,CBT)是要改变脑卒中患者的认知活动过程,指出其错误的思维方法和由此产生的错误观念,启发和引导进行合乎理性的逻辑思维,放弃对自身破坏性的观念和情绪,重新建立神经环路,从而达到矫正认知行为的目的。

平衡心理治疗(balancing psychotherapy,BPT)是一种建立在东方哲学体系上的,整合多种心理流派的治疗取向。它运用心身平衡理论和方法打通思维阻塞,为 PSD 患者分析病因,看清使得内稳态失衡的思维阻塞内容,再提供思路,引导 PSD 患者对问题作全方位、本质的认识,然后从现实生活中举出相应事例加以比较,让患者以出离心观察自我、重塑认知,最后与其探讨如何行动,最终使内部平衡重建。心理治疗可用于轻、中度抑郁的辅助治疗。

5.4 其他治疗

音乐治疗、针灸治疗[109]、太极拳、高压氧[110]等均可用于 PSD 的治疗,但目前尚缺乏设计良好的随机对照研究结果支持其疗效。

6 PSD 的预防性治疗

早期预防性治疗能有效减少 PSD 的发生并对神经功能恢复起较大促进作用[111]。抗抑郁剂及心理治疗均可提高卒中患者的日常生活能力、认知功能及降低病死率[112]。

预防性使用抗抑郁剂可以显著减少 PSD 的发生率。抗抑郁剂特别是 SSRIs 在预防 PSD 的发生及提高卒中后患者的预后中起到了重要的作用[113]。

乌灵胶囊对 PSD 也有一定的预防作用,可以降低 PSD 发生率、延缓 PSD 发生时间并减轻 PSD 严重程度[114]。

运动再学习技术(motor relearning programme,MRP)把中枢神经系统损伤后运动功能的恢复训练当作是一种再学习或再训练的过程,在卒中常规治疗、药物治疗的基础上进行早期 MRP 训练能明显降低 PSD 发生率[115]。

由社区健康专业人员对患者进行电话访问,撰写健康教育材料、家访与健康专业者联系,以及健康服务的转诊能够有效地降低 PSD 的严重程度,并提高患者的生活质量[116]。

PSD 的发生与生物、心理、社会因素有着密切的关系。认知行为治疗、问题解决疗法以及家庭治疗对脑卒中患者有效,且可提高 PSD 的认知功能和生活质量[117]。

总之,早期预防对于减少 PSD 发生,促进功能恢复起着重要作用。但关于预防的策略和时间目前仍有较多争议,提倡对于卒中患者及早进行生活方式宣教,心理疏导和干预等非药物预防为宜[116,117]。

7 PSD 的护理

PSD 患者的功能失调问题,使其需要更多的护理措施,护理人员和家庭照料者在 PSD 患者恢复中扮演重要角色[118]，而他们对疾病的理解也是影响疾病发展、预后的重要因素[119]。同时，护理人员所承受的照顾压力和自身的精神健康也会影 PSD 患者的疾病恢复[120, 121]。因此，护理及心理干预对急性期及恢复期 PSD 患者均十分重要。

良好的护理措施应该以全面的护理评估为基础，这包括了对躯体状况、心理状况及相关风险因素的评估。护理工作要提供必要的情感支持，减少陌生环境导致的不安全感，使患者尽快适应。可在 PSD 早期引入家属陪护的亲情化护理管理措施。

基础护理工作包括提供舒适的环境、提供恰当的个人生活护理、及时补充营养并创造一个好的睡眠环境保证充分的睡眠。冷漠和嗜睡是导致卒中患者康复训练减少的重要原因[122]，护理人员应该帮助患者克服卒中带来的此类问题，让患者尽快进行卒中后的康复训练。有效的床旁训练可改善 PSD 患者情绪并促进躯体功能恢复，提高生活质量[123]。

心理护理主要通过促进健康、减少应激、提高应对技巧发挥作用[124]。PSD 患者面对躯体功能障碍时容易产生挫败感[125]，因此，护理人员要尊重并关心患者，帮助患者了解疾病、建立信心并适当给予支持性心理治疗。

全程健康教育对减轻 PSD 病人的抑郁症状有明显改善效果[126]。全程一体化健康教育包括：急性期（1～2 周）给予支持性心理治疗；稳定期（3～4 周）以集体宣教方式为主，可采用多媒体健康教育方式；康复期（4～6 周）巩固疗效，预防复发，鼓励患者重返社会，承担工作、生活的重任[127]。

另外，护士应结合患者的具体情况和需求，制定个体化、全程护理方案。出院前实施出院健康指导，出院后 1～2 周电话回访，再次进行答疑及健康教育。护士对患者实施全程健康教育，能够促进患者自觉建立健康的行为模式，消除不良情绪，提高治疗信心，从而全身心投入治疗及康复中，最终减轻 PSD 症状。

8 PSD 的诊断和治疗流程(见图 2)

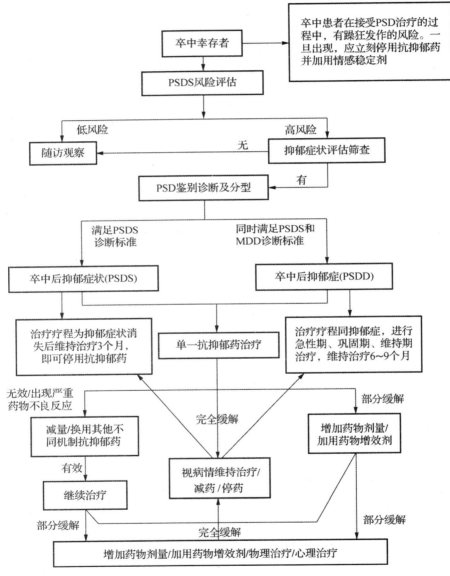

图 2 PSD 诊治流程图

9 PSD 的人群防治及管理

医务人员培训：在各级卫生部门和政策的支持下,积极进行医务人员培训对于可持续开展 PSD 的防治极为重要。以各地精神卫生医疗机构为主要培训基地,对各级综合性医院、专科医院、乡镇社区卫生院和护理院中的精神科医师、非精神科医师、心理咨询师、心理治疗师、医疗护理人员等进行 PSD 诊治的系统培训,建立一支由各级医疗卫生部门组成的可用人力资源、能广泛和有效开展 PSD 防治的精神卫生基础服务队伍。

精神卫生的健康教育：通过报告会、专题讲座、家庭访谈、宣传单、壁报栏、科普文章、电台广播等口头、文字、形象宣传等方式,开发和动员各种媒体的广泛参与,扩大宣传效应,提高社会人群对 PSD 的知晓率、识别率和就治率。

建立评估监测系统：对患者心身状态、功能障碍和生活质量等方面进行综合性监测和安全评估,及时发现高危人群,进行心理社会干预。对住院患者进行心身联络会诊服务,为其他科室(如神经内科、康复科)的 PSD 患者提供诊断、治疗处理建议和咨询服务。

建立良好医患关系及三级预防：通过医患之间的沟通,建立巩固良好的医患关系、提高防治依从性是提高治疗效果和治愈率的有效途径。此外,由于精神疾病治疗模式的局限性,有效实施和进行三级预防是减少精神行为障碍所致的残疾、减轻家庭和社会负担的有效策略。其中一级预防即病因预防,通过最积极、最主动的预防措施减少 PSD 的发生;二级预防的重点是早期发现、早期诊断、早期治疗,争取良好预后;三级预防的要点是防止疾病复发,做好康复训练,最大限度地促进患者社会功能恢复,提高患者生活质量。

参考文献

[1] Gainotti G, Azzoni A, Marra C. Frequency, phenomenology and anatomical-clinical

correlates of major post-stroke depression [J]. Br J Psychiatry, 1999, 175: 163 - 167.

[2] Lipsey JR, Spencer WC, Rabins PV, Robinson RG. Phenomenological comparison of poststroke depression and functional depression [J]. Am J Psychiatry, 1986, 143(4): 527 - 529.

[3] Fedoroff JP, Starkstein SE, Parikh RM, Price TR, Robinson RG. Are depressive symptoms nonspecific in patients with acute stroke? [J]. Am J Psychiatry, 1991, 148(9): 1172 - 1176.

[4] Jiao JT, Cheng C, Ma YJ, Huang J, Dai MC, Jiang C, Wang C, Shao JF. Association between inflammatory cytokines and the risk of post-stroke depression, and the effect of depression on outcomes of patients with ischemic stroke in a 2-year prospective study [J]. Exp Ther Med, 2016, 12: 1591 - 1598.

[5] Pompili M, Venturini P, Campi S, Seretti ME, Montebovi F, Lamis DA, Serafini G, Amore M, Girardi P. Do stroke patients have an increased risk of developing suicidal ideation or dying by suicide? An overview of the current literature [J]. CNS Neurosci Ther, 2012, 18: 711 - 721.

[6] Robert G, Robinson MD, Ricardo E, Jorge MD. Post-Stroke Depression: A Review [J]. Am J Psychiatry, 2016, 173(3): 221 - 31.

[7] Hackett ML, Pickles K. Part I: frequency of depression after stroke: an updated systematic review and meta-analysis of observational studies [J]. Int J Stroke, 2014, 9(8):1017 - 1025.

[8] Ferro JM, Caeiro L, Santos C. Poststroke emotional and behavior impairment: a narrative review [J]. Cerebrovasc Dis, 2009, 27(suppl1): 197 - 203.

[9] 游林林. 社会心理风险因素与缺血性脑卒中后抑郁心理生理机制的关联研究[D]. 苏州大学, 2016.

[10] Shi Y, Xiang Y, Yang Y, Zhang N, Wang S, Ungvari GS, et al. Depression after minor stroke: Prevalence and predictors [J]. J Psychosom Res. 2015, 79(2):143 - 147.

[11] Sun N, Li QJ, Lv DM, Man J, Liu XS, Sun ML. A survey on 465 patients with post-stroke depression in China [J]. Arch Psychiatr Nurs. 2014: 28(6):368

- 371.

[12] Gordon WA, Hibbard MR. Poststroke depression: an examination of the literature [J]. Arch Phys Med Rehabil, 1997, 78(6): 658 - 663.

[13] Tang WK, Chan SS, Chiu HF, Ungvari GS, Wong KS, Kwok TC, Mok V, Wong KT, Richards PS, Ahuja AT. Poststroke depression in Chinese patients: frequency, psychosocial, clinical, and radiological determinants [J]. J Geriatr Psychiatry Neurol, 2005, 18(1): 45 - 51.

[14] Andersen G, Vestergaard K, Riis J, Lauritzen L. Incidence of post-stroke depression during the first year in a large unselected stroke population determined using a valid standardized rating scale [J]. Acta Psychiatr Scand, 1994, 90(3): 190 - 195.

[15] Zhang T, Wang C, Liu L, Zhao X, Xue J, Zhou Y, Wang Y, Wang Y. A prospective cohort study of the incidence and determinants of post-stroke depression among the mainland Chinese patients [J]. Neurol Res, 2010, 32(4): 347 - 352.

[16] Zhang N, Wang CX, Wang AX, Bai Y, Zhou Y, Wang YL, Zhang T, Zhou J, Yu X, Sun XY, Liu ZR, Zhao XQ, Wang YJ, on behalf of the Prospective Cohort study on Incidence and Outcome of Patients with Poststroke Depression in China (PRIOD) Investigators. Time course of depression and one-year prognosis of patients with stroke in mainland China [J]. CNS Neurosci Ther, 2012, 18(6): 475 - 481.

[17] Hackett ML, Yapa C, Parag V, Anderson CS. Frequency of depression after stroke: a systematic review of observational studies [J]. Stroke, 2005, 36(6): 1330 - 1340.

[18] Chemerinski E, Robinson RG. The neuropsychiatry of stroke [J]. Psychosomatics, 2000, 41(1): 5 - 14.

[19] Morris PL, Robinson RG, Raphael B. Prevalence and course of depressive disorders in hospitalized stroke patients [J]. Int J Psychiatry Med, 1990, 20(4): 349 - 364.

[20] Chemerinski E, Robinson RG, and Kosier JT. Improved recovery in activities of daily living associated with remission of poststroke depression [J]. Stroke, 2001,

32(1)：113－117.

[21] 范清雨,屈秋民,张虹,刘璟洁,郭峰,乔晋. 卒中后认知功能变化规律及其影响因素分析 [J]. 中华内科杂志, 2011, 50 (9)：750－753.

[22] Fultz NH, Ofstedal MB, Herzog AR, Wallace RB. Additive and interactive effects of comorbid physical and mental conditions on functional health [J]. J Aging Health, 2003, 15(3)：465－481.

[23] Yang Y, Shi YZ, Zhang N, Wang S, Ungvari GS, Ng CH, et al. The Disability Rate of 5-Year Post-Stroke and Its Correlation Factors：A National Survey in China. PLoS One. 2016; 11 (11)：e0165341.

[24] Kishi Y, Robinson RG, Kosier JT. Suicidal plans in patients with stroke：comparison between acute-onset and delayed-onset suicidal plans [J]. Int Psychogeriatr, 1996, 8(4)：623－634.

[25] Yang Y, Shi YZ, Zhang N, Wang S, Ungvari GS, Ng CH, et al. Suicidal ideation at 1-year post-stroke：A nationwide survey in China [J]. Gen Hosp Psychiatry. 2017, 44：38－42.

[26] Feigin VL, Krishnamurthi RV, Parmar P, Norrving B, Mensah GA, Bennett DA, Barker-Collo S, Moran AE, Sacco RL, Truelsen T, Davis S, Pandian JD, Naghavi M, Forouzanfar MH, Nguyen G, Johnson CO, Vos T, Meretoja A, Murray CJ, Roth GA, GBD 2013 Writing Group and GBD 2013 Stroke Panel Experts Group. Update on the Global Burden of Ischemic and Hemorrhagic Stroke in 1990—2013：The GBD 2013 Study [J]. Neuroepidemiology, 2015, 45(3)：161－176.

[27] Yang G, Wang Y, Zeng Y, Gao GF, Liang X, Zhou M, Wan X, Yu S, Jiang Y, Naghavi M, Vos T, Wang H, Lopez AD, Murray CJ. Rapid health transition in China, 1990—2010：findings from the Global Burden of Disease Study 2010 [J]. Lancet, 2013, 381(9882)：1987－2015.

[28] 刘克军,王梅. 我国慢性病直接经济负担研究 [J]. 中国卫生经济, 2005,24(10)：77－80.

[29] Han YH, Liu YL, Zhang XL, Tam W, Mao J, Lopez V. Chinese family caregivers of stroke survivors：Determinants of caregiving burden within the first six months [J]. J Clin Nurs. 2017;26(23-24):4558－4566.

[30] Paolucci S. Advances in antidepressants for treating post-stroke depression [J]. Expert Opin Pharmacother. 2017，18(10)：1011－1017.

[31] Verdelho A，Hénon H，Lebert F，Pasquier F，Leys D. Depressive symptoms after stroke and relationship with dementia：A three-year follow-up study [J]. Neurology，2004，62(6)：905－911.

[32] Hadidi N，Treat-Jacobson DJ，Lindquist R. Poststroke depression and functional outcome：a critical review of literature [J]. Heart Lung，2009，38(2)：151－162.

[33] Zhang WN，Pan YH，Wang XY，Zhao Y. A prospective study of the incidence and correlated factors of post-stroke depression in China [J]. PLoS One，2013，8(11)：e78981.

[34] De Ryck A，Brouns R，Fransen E，Geurden M，Van Gestel G，Wilssens I，De Ceulaer L，Mariën P，De Deyn PP，Engelborghs S. A prospective study on the prevalence and risk factors of poststroke depression [J]. Cerebrovasc Dis Extra，2013，3(1)：1－13.

[35] Göthe F，Enache D，Wahlund LO，Winblad B，Crisby M，Lökk J，Aarsland D. Cerebrovascular diseases and depression：epidemiology，mechanisms and treatment [J]. Panminerva Med，2012，54(3)：161－170.

[36] Townend BS，Whyte S，Desborough T，Crimmins D，Markus R，Levi C，Sturm JW. Longitudinal prevalence and determinants of early mood disorder post-stroke [J]. J Clin Neurosci，2007，14(5)：429－434.

[37] 李丹. 首次脑卒中后抑郁相关因素分析[D]. 内蒙古民族大学，2013.

[38] Storor DL，Byrne GJ. Pre-morbid personality and depression following stroke [J]. Int Psychogeriatr，2006，18(3)：457－469.

[39] 梁翠萍，王欣森，徐金秀，王贺波，李振芳. 脑卒中后抑郁与心理社会因素的关系研究 [J]. 中国临床心理学杂志，2005，13(4)：470－471，473.

[40] Kohen R，Cain KC，Mitchell PH，Becker KJ，Buzaitis A，Millard SP，Navaja GP，Teri L，Tirschwell D，Veith R. Association of serotonin transporter gene polymorphisms with poststroke depression [J]. Arch Gen Psychiatry，2008，65(11)：1296－1302.

[41] 陈爱敏. 5-羟色胺 1A 受体、G 蛋白 β 白亚基基因多态性与卒中后抑郁的相关性研

究［D］. 南方医科大学，2011.

[42] 陈翠，刘振华，陈爱敏，赵连旭. 5-羟色胺 2A 受体 T102C 基因多态性与卒中后抑郁的关联研究［J］. 中华神经医学杂志，2011，10(11)：1119－1121.

[43] Kim JM，Stewart R，Bae KY，Kim SW，Kang HJ，Shin IS，Kim JT，Park MS，Kim MK，Park SW，Kim YH，Kim JK，Cho KH，Yoon JS. Serotonergic and BDNF genes and risk of depression after stroke［J］. J Affect Disord，2012，136(3)：833－840.

[44] 曹琳，刘振华，赵连旭. 血浆同型半胱氨酸和 MTHFR 基因多态性与卒中后抑郁的相关性分析［J］. 广东医学，2010，31(22)：2946－2949.

[45] 蔡卫卫. 多巴胺代谢系统儿茶酚氧位甲基转移酶、多巴胺转运体基因多态性与卒中后抑郁的相关性分析［D］. 南方医科大学，2011.

[46] Kim JM，Stewart R，Kim SW，Shin IS，Kim JT，Park MS，Park SW，Kim YH，Cho KH，Yoon JS. Associations of cytokine gene polymorphisms with post-stroke depression［J］. World J Biol Psychiatry，2012，13(8)：579－587.

[47] 贺丽敏. 卒中后抑郁与 CREB1 基因多态性相关分析［D］. 南方医科大学，2010.

[48] Zhao L，Li H，Guo R，Ma T，Hou R，Ma X，Du Y. miR-137，a new target for post-stroke depression?［J］. Neural Regen Res，2013，8(26)：2441－2448.

[49] Bryer JB，Starkstein SE，Votypka V，Parikh RM，Price TR，Robinson RG. Reduction of CSF monoamine metabolites in poststroke depression：a preliminary report［J］. J Neuropsychiatry Clin Neurosci，1992，4(4)：440－442.

[50] Ghika-Schmid F，Bogousslavsky J. Affective disorders following stroke［J］. Eur Neurol，1997，38(2)：75－81.

[51] Glodzik-Sobanska L，Slowik A，McHugh P，Sobiecka B，Kozub J，Rich KE，Urbanik A，Szczudlik A. Single voxel proton magnetic resonance spectroscopy in post-stroke depression［J］. Psychiatry Res，2006，148(2-3)：111－120.

[52] Maines MD. Zinc. Protoporphyrin is a selective inhibitor of heme oxygenase activity in the neonatal rat［J］. Biochim Biophys Acta，1981，673(3)：339－350.

[53] Kuo HK，Yen CJ，Chang CH，Kuo CK，Chen JH，Sorond F. Relation of C-reactive protein to stroke，cognitive disorders，and depression in the general population：systematic review and meta-analysis［J］. Lancet Neurol，2005，4(6)：371

－380.

[54] Paolucci S, Autonucci G, Grasso MG, Morelli D, Troisi E, Coiro P, De Angelis D, Rizzi F, Bragoni M. Poststroke depression, antidepressant treatment and reha-bilitation result. A case-control study [J]. Cerebrovasc Dis Extra, 2001, 12: 264 －271.

[55] 熊光润，赵凌云，毛建平. 老年期女性脑卒中后抑郁患者下丘脑-垂体-性腺轴功能变化的研究 [J]. 神经疾病与精神卫生，2007,7(3)：180－182.

[56] Yang L, Zhang Z, Sun D, Xu Z, Yuan Y, Zhang X, Li L. Low serum BDNF may indicate the development of PSD in patients with acute ischemic stroke [J]. Int J Geriatr Psychiatry, 2011, 26(5): 495－502.

[57] Zhu L, Han B, Wang L, Chang Y, Ren W, Gu Y, Yan M, Wu C, Zhang XY, He J. The association between serum ferritin levels and post-stroke depression [J]. J Affect Disord, 2016, 190: 98－102.

[58] Tang CZ, Zhang YL, Wang WS, Li WG, Shi JP. Elevated serum levels of neop-terin at admission predicts depression after acute ischemic stroke: a 6-month fol-low-up study[J]. Mol Neurobiol, 2016, 53(5): 3194－3204.

[59] Kim JS, Choi-Kwon S. Poststroke depression and emotional incontinence: correla-tion with lesion location [J]. Neurology, 2000, 54(9): 1805－1810.

[60] Hama S, Yamashita H, Shigenobu M, Watanabe A, Kurisu K, Yamawaki S, Kitaoka T. Post-stroke affective or apathetic depression and lesion location: left frontal lobe and bilateral basal ganglia [J]. Eur Arch Psychiatry Clin Neurosci, 2007, 257(3): 149－152.

[61] Robinson RG, Kubos KL, Starr LB, Rao K, Price TR. Mood disorders in stroke patients Importance of location of lesion [J]. Brain: a journal of neurology. 1984, 107 (Pt 1):81－93.

[62] Wei N, Yong W, Li X, Zhou Y, Deng M, Zhu H, Jin H. Post-stroke depression and lesion location: a systematic review [J]. J Neurol, 2015, 262(1): 81－90.

[63] Tang WK, Chen YK, Lu JY, Chu WC, Mok VC, Ungvari GS, Wong KS. White matter hyperintensities in post-stroke depression: a case control study [J]. J Neu-rol Neurosurg Psychiatry, 2010, 81(12): 1312－1315.

[64] de Man-van Ginkel JM, Hafsteinsdóttir TB, Lindeman E, Ettema RG, Grobbee DE, Schuurmans MJ. In-hospital risk prediction for post-stroke depression: development and validation of the Post-stroke Depression Prediction Scale [J]. Stroke, 2013, 44(9): 2441 – 2445.

[65] Jiang XG, Lin Y, Li YS. Correlative study on risk factors of depression among acute stroke patients [J]. Eur Rev Med Pharmacol Sci, 2014, 18(9): 1315 – 1323.

[66] Wang LR, Tao Y, Wang H, Zhou HD, Fu XY. Association of post stroke depression with social factors, insomnia, and neurological status in Chinese elderly population [J]. Neurol Sci. 2016 Aug;37(8):1305 – 1310.

[67] Schulz R, Beach SR, Ives DG, Martire LM, Ariyo AA, Kop WJ. Association between depression and mortality in older adults: the Cardiovascular Health Study [J]. Arch Intern Med, 2000, 160(12): 1761 – 1768.

[68] Aben I, Verhey F, Strik J, Lousberg R, Lodder J, Honig A. A comparative study into the one year cumulative incidence of depression after stroke and myocardial infarction [J]. J Neurol Neurosurg Psychiatry, 2003, 74(5): 581 – 585.

[69] Brott T, Adams HP Jr, Olinger CP, Marler JR, Barsan WG, Biller J, Spilker J, Holleran R, Eberle R, Hertzberg V, Rorick M, Moomaw CJ, Walker M. Measurements of acute cerebral infarction: a clinical examination scale [J]. Stroke, 1989, 20(7): 864 – 870.

[70] Rankin J. Cerebral vascular accidents in patients over the age of 60. II. Prognosis [J]. Scott Med J, 1957, 2(5): 200 – 215.

[71] Mahoney FI, Barthel DW. Functional evaluation: the Barthel Index. Md State Med J, 1965, 14: 61 – 65.

[72] Zung W. A self-rating depression scale. Arch Gen Psychiatry, 1965, 12: 63 – 70.

[73] Beck AT, Ward CH, Mendelson M, Mock J, Erbaugh J. An inventory for measuring depression [J]. Arch Gen Psychiatry, 1961, 4: 561 – 571.

[74] Wang W, Bian Q, Zhao Y, Li X, Wang W, Du J, Zhang G, Zhou Q, Zhao M. Reliability and validity of the Chinese version of the Patient Health Questionnaire (PHQ-9) in the general population [J]. Gen Hosp Psychiatry, 2014, 36(5): 539 – 544.

[75]　Snaith RP, Zigmond AS. The hospital anxiety and depression scale [J]. Br Med J (Clin Res Ed), 1986, 292(6516): 344.

[76]　Radloff LS. The CES-D scale A self-report depression scale for research in the general population [J]. Appl Psychol Meas, 1977, 1(3): 385 – 401.

[77]　Hamilton M. A rating scale for depression [J]. J Neurol Neurosurg Psychiatry, 1960, 23(1): 56 – 62.

[78]　Montgomery SA, Asberg M. A new depression scale designed to be sensitive to change [J]. Br J Psychiatry, 1979, 134(4): 382 – 389.

[79]　Yue Y, Liu R, Lu J, Wang XJ, Zhang SN, Wu AQ, Wang Q, Yuan YG. Reliability and validity of a new post-stroke depression scale in Chinese population [J]. J Affect Disord, 2015, 174: 317 – 323.

[80]　Williams LS, Brizendine EJ, Plue L, Bakas T, Tu WZ, Hendrie H, Kroenke K. Performance of the PHQ-9 as a screening tool for depression after stroke [J]. Stroke, 2005, 36(3): 635 – 638.

[81]　American Psychiatric Association. Diagnostic and Statistical Manual of Mental Disorders (DSM-IV). Washington: American Psychiatric Association, 2013.

[82]　Yue Y, Liu R, Cao Y, Wu Y, Zhang S, Li H, Zhu J, Jiang W, Wu A, Yuan Y. New opinion on the subtypes of poststroke depression in Chinese stroke survivors [J]. Neuropsychiatr Dis Treat, 2017, 13: 707 – 713.

[83]　Withall A, Brodaty H, Altendorf A, Sachdev PS. A longitudinal study examining the independence of apathy and depression after stroke: the Sydney Stroke Study [J]. Int Psychogeriatr, 2011, 23(2): 264 – 273.

[84]　Ishizaki J, Mimura M. Dysthymia and apathy: diagnosis and treatment [J]. Depress Res Treat, 2011: 893 – 905.

[85]　Campbell Burton CA, Murray J, Holmes J, Astin F, Greenwood D, Knapp P. Frequency of anxiety after stroke: a systematic review andmeta-analysis of observational studies [J]. Int J Stroke, 2013, 8(7): 545 – 559.

[86]　Schottke H, Giabbiconi CM. Post-stroke depression and post-stroke anxiety: prevalence and predictors [J]. Int Psychogeriatr, 2015, 27(11): 1805 – 1812.

[87]　Staub F, Bogousslavsky J. Fatigue after stroke: a major but neglected issue [J].

Cerebrovasc Dis，2001，12(2)：75－81.

[88] Almeida OP，Xiao J. Mortality associated with incident mental health disorders after stroke [J]. Aust N Z J Psychiatry，2007，41(3)：274－281.

[89] Xu XM 1，Zou DZ，Shen LY，Liu Y，Zhou XY，Pu JC，Dong MX，Wei YD. Efficacy and feasibility of antidepressant treatment in patients with post-stroke depression [J]. Med，2016，95：45(e5349).

[90] Horváth S，Karányi Z，Harcos P，Nagy Z，Németh G，Andor G. Clinical effectiveness and safety of paroxetine in post-stroke depression：results from a phase 4，open label，multicenter clinical trial with 26 weeks of follow-up [J]. Orv Hetil，2006，147(50)：2397－2404.

[91] Andersen G，Vestergaard K，Lauritzen L. Effective treatment of poststroke depression with the selective serotonin reuptake inhibitor citalopram [J]. Stroke，1994，25(6)：1099－1104.

[92] 武文珺，王怀海，彭正午，王莹，张雅红，何宏，谭庆荣. 4 种 SSRI 类抗抑郁药物治疗卒中后抑郁的疗效及对生活质量的影响 [J]. 神经疾病与精神卫生，2013，13(1)：16－19.

[93] Spalletta G，Caltagirone C. Sertraline treatment of post-stroke major depression：an open study in patients with moderate to severe symptoms [J]. Funct Neurol，2003，18(4)：227－232.

[94] Sunami E，Usuda K，Nishiyama Y，Otori T，Katsura K，Katayama Y. A preliminary study of fluvoxamine maleate on depressive state and serum melatonin levels in patients after cerebral infarction [J]. Intern Med，2012，51(10)：1187－1193.

[95] Niedermaier N，Bohrer E，Schulte K，Schlattmann P，Heuser I. Prevention and treatment of poststroke depression with mirtazapine in patients with acute stroke [J]. J Clin Psychiatry，2004，65(12)：1619－1623.

[96] Yi ZM，Liu F，Zhai SD. Fluoxetine for the prophylaxis of poststroke depression in patients with stroke：a meta-analysis [J]. Int J Clin Pract，2010，64(9)：1310－1317.

[97] Smith D，Dempster C，Glanville J，Freemantle N，Anderson I. Efficacy and tolerability of venlafaxine compared with selective serotonin reuptake inhibitors and other antidepres-

sants: a meta-analysis [J]. Br J Psychiatry, 2002, 180: 396 - 404.

[98] Tan S, Huang XY, Ding L, Hong H. Efficacy and Safety of Citalopram in Treating Post-Stroke Depression: A Meta-Analysis [J]. Eur Neurol 2015; 74: 188 - 201.

[99] 孙新字，陈爱琴，许秀峰，张宏根，唐启盛，张鸿燕. 舒肝解郁胶囊治疗轻中度抑郁症的随机双盲安慰剂对照研究[J]. 中国新药杂志，2009，18（05）：413 - 416，457.

[100] 汪亚群，宋水江，江霞. 乌灵胶囊合左洛复治疗脑卒中后抑郁的临床研究 [J]. 浙江中医杂志，2007，42（4）：202 - 203.

[101] Fruehwald S, Gatterbauer E, Rehak P, Baumhackl U. Early fluoxetine treatment of post-stroke depression—a three-month double-blind placebo-controlled study with an open-label long-term follow up [J]. J Neurol, 2003, 250(3): 347 - 351.

[102] Gao J, Lin MQ, Zhao JH, Bi SW, Ni ZY, Shang XL. Different interventions for post-ischaemic stroke depression in different time periods: A single-blind randomized controlled trial with stratification by time after stroke [J]. Clin Rehabil, 2017 Jan;31(1):71 - 81.

[103] Hebert D, Lindsay MP, McIntyre A, Kirton A, Rumney PG, Bagg S, et al. Canadian stroke best practice recommendations: Stroke rehabilitation practice guidelines, update 2015 [J]. Int J Stroke, 2016, 11: 459 - 484.

[104] Jorge RE, Robinson RG, Tateno A, Narushima K, Acion L, Moser D, Arndt S, Chemerinski E. Repetitive transcranial magnetic stimulation as treatment of poststroke depression: a preliminary study [J]. Biol Psychiatry, 2004, 55(4): 398 - 405.

[105] Shen X, Liu M, Cheng Y, Jia C, Pan X, Gou Q, Liu X, Cao H, Zhang L. Repetitive transcranial magnetic stimulation for the treatment of post-stroke depression: A systematic review and meta-analysis of randomized controlled clinical trials [J]. J Affect Disord. 2017; 211: 65 - 74.

[106] Currier MB, Murray GB, and Welch CC. Electroconvulsive therapy for post-stroke depressed geriatric patients [J]. J Neuropsychiatry Clin Neurosci, 1992, 4 (2): 140 - 144.

[107] Friedland JF, McColl M. Social support intervention after stroke: results of a

randomized trial [J]. Arch Phys Med Rehabil, 1992, 73(6): 573 - 581.

[108] Nicholl CR, Lincoln NB, Muncaster K, Thomas S. Cognitions and post-stroke depression [J]. Br J Clin Psychol, 2002, 41(Pt 3): 221 - 231.

[109] Zhang ZJ, Chen HY, Yip KC, Ng R, Wong VT. The effectiveness and safety of acupuncture therapy in depressive disorders: systematic review and meta-analysis [J]. J Affect Disord, 2010, 124(1-2): 9 - 21.

[110] Yan D, Shan J, Ze Y, Zeng XY, Hu XH. The effects of combined hyperbaric oxygen therapy on patients with post-stroke depression [J]. J Phys Ther Sci, 2015, 27 (5): 1295 - 1297.

[111] 王锋. 早期预防卒中后抑郁对急性脑卒中患者康复治疗的影响 [J]. 中国现代药物应用, 2013, 7(20): 98 - 99.

[112] Ramasubbu R. Therapy for prevention of post-stroke depression [J]. Expert Opin Pharmacother, 2011, 12(14): 2177 - 2187.

[113] Flaster M, Sharma A, Rao M. Poststroke depression: a review emphasizing the role of prophylactic treatment and synergy with treatment for motor recovery [J]. Top Stroke Rehabil, 2013, 20(2): 139 - 150.

[114] 朱瑾, 胡春梅, 郭思思, 王锋, 周叶, 张素雅. 乌灵胶囊辅助治疗对卒中后抑郁一级预防作用的临床观察 [J]. 中国中西医结合杂志, 2014, 34(6): 676 - 679.

[115] Langhammer B, Stanghelle JK. Bobath or motor relearning programme? A comparison of two different approaches of physiotherapy in stroke rehabilitation: a randomized controlled study [J]. Clin Rehabil, 2000, 14(4): 361 - 369.

[116] Graven C, Brock K, Hill K, Ames D, Cotton S, Joubert L. From rehabilitation to recovery: protocol for a randomised controlled trial evaluating a goal-based intervention to reduce depression and facilitate participation post-stroke [J]. BMC Neurol, 2011, 11: 73.

[117] Desmond DW, Remien RH, Moroney JT, Stern Y, Sano M, Williams JB. Ischemic stroke and depression [J]. J Int Neuropsychol Soc, 2003, 9(3): 429 - 439.

[118] Clark PC, Dunbar SB, Aycock DM, Courtney E, Wolf SL. Caregiver perspectives of memory and behavior changes in stroke survivors [J]. Rehabil Nurs, 2006, 31(1): 26 - 32.

[119]　Bennett B. How nurses in a stroke rehabilitation unit attempt to meet the psycho-logical needs of patients who become depressed following a stroke [J]. J Adv Nurs，1996，23(2)：314－321.

[120]　Evans RL，Bishop DS，Haselkorn JK. Factors predicting satisfactory home care after stroke [J]. Arch Phys Med Rehabil，1991，72(2)：144－147.

[121]　Suh M，Kim K，Kim I，Cho N，Choi H，Noh S. Caregiver's burden，depression and support as predictors of post-stroke depression：a cross-sectional survey [J]. Int J Nurs Stud，2005，42(6)：611－618.

[122]　Harris AL，Elder J，Schiff ND，Victor JD，Goldfine AM. Post-stroke apathy and hypersomnia lead to worse outcomes from acute rehabilitation [J]. Transl Stroke Res，2014，5(2)：292－300.

[123]　Kang JH，Park RY，Lee SJ，Kim JY，Yoon SR，Jung KI. The effect of bedside exercise program on stroke patients with Dysphagia [J]. Ann Rehabil Med，2012，36(4)：512－520.

[124]　Eldred C，Sykes C. Psychosocial interventions for carers of survivors of stroke：a systematic review of interventions based on psychological principles and theoreti-cal frameworks [J]. Br J Health Psychol，2008，13(Pt 3)：563－581.

[125]　Kouwenhoven SE，Kirkevold M，Engedal K，Kim HS. 'Living a life in shades of grey'：experiencing depressive symptoms in the acute phase after stroke [J]. J Adv Nurs，2012，68(8)：1726－1737.

[126]　杜芳，李遵清，于青，阮玖琼. 全程一体化健康教育改善抑郁障碍患者抑郁情绪及心理障碍的效果 [J]. 中华行为医学与脑科学杂志，2011,20(5)：434－436.

[作者及发表刊物(本文已以英文发表)：

Fuying Zhao，Yingying Yue，Lei Li，Senyang Lang，Mingwei Wang，Xiangdong Du，Yunlong Deng，Aiqin Wu，and Yonggui Yuan*. Clinical practice guidelines for post-stroke depression in China，Rev Bras Psiquiatr，2018，doi：10. 1590/1516-4446-2017-2343. （Epub ahead of print)]

心身医学研究用诊断标准(DCPR)简介

摘要：1995 年国际心身医学研究小组首次提出心身医学研究用诊断标准（DCPR），以弥补美国精神障碍诊断与统计手册第四版（DSM-Ⅳ）对心身疾病诊断的不足。2017 年该小组对 DCPR 进行了修订并增加 2 个条目内容（适应负荷与疑病症）。我们结合中国当前临床实际，在新版 DCPR 的基础上进一步修订，增加 4 个条目内容（神经质、逛医行为、体象障碍、重大疾病/手术后的躯体不适），并将疑病症改为疑病观念，最终形成三方面共 18 项诊断条目的中国版心身医学研究用诊断标准（CDCPR）。

关键词：DCPR；CDCPR

一、前言

心身医学是一个研究生物、心理和社会因素在调节健康和疾病平衡过程中相互作用的广泛性交叉学科[1]。过去的几十年，人们对与躯体疾病的易损性、治疗和预后的密切相关的可调节的心理因素的评估也日益关注。依赖于心身医学相关的科研成果在很多重要杂志期刊，如《Psychotherapy and Psychosomatics》、《Psychosomatic Medicine》、《Psychosomatics》和《Journal of Psychosomatic Research》大量发表，心身医学形成了一个有一定影响力的知识体系。这个知识体系的应用产生出了一些分支学科：心理肿瘤学、心理肾脏病学、心理神经内分泌学、心理神经胃肠病学、行为心脏病学、心理免疫学、心理皮肤病学等等，而这些学科的出现及发展反过来又促进了医学期刊、临床服务以及科学的发展[2]。临床上，心身疾病很常见，虽然并未达到精神障碍的诊断标准，却显著影响着患者的生命质量以及疾病的转归和预后，且其发病率较精神疾病更高。然而，临床医生大多使用美国的精神障碍诊断与统计手册第四版

(DSM-Ⅳ)进行诊断,而心身疾病的发病机制和临床症状特征与精神障碍不同,采用精神障碍分类诊断标准会导致大量达不到诊断标准却存在社会心理易感因素或躯体化症状的患者难以得到有效的关注。可以说采用这种诊断模式几乎无法对当前心身医学的临床实践产生实质性的帮助[3]。而在科研上,研究者也往往采用不同的诊断工具,使得研究结果同质性较差,同时这种分类诊断模式也不利于研究者间的交流。

二、1995 年版心身医学研究用诊断标准

为了补充 DSM 诊断系统临床应用的不足,1995 年国际心身医学研究小组提出心身医学研究用诊断标准(Diagnostic Criteria for Psychosomatic Research,DCPR),这是一个简单、可靠且有效的定式访谈工具,包含了十二个综合征,可分为两组:(1) 关注心理因素对健康的影响,共四个综合征,包括述情障碍、A 型行为、沮丧和易激惹,这四个症状更好地替代了 DSM-Ⅳ 中的"影响医学情况的心理因素";(2) 关注异常疾病行为,共八个,包括疾病恐惧、死亡恐惧、健康焦虑和疾病否认、继发于精神障碍的功能性躯体症状、持续性躯体化、转换症状及周年反应,这八个综合征取代和扩大了 DSM 中"躯体形式障碍"这一章节(见图 1)。

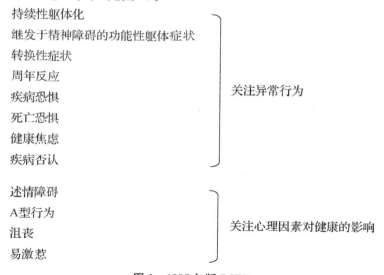

持续性躯体化
继发于精神障碍的功能性躯体症状
转换性症状
周年反应
疾病恐惧
死亡恐惧
健康焦虑
疾病否认
} 关注异常行为

述情障碍
A型行为
沮丧
易激惹
} 关注心理因素对健康的影响

图 1　1995 年版 DCPR

DCPR 通过将影响躯体疾病治疗和预后的心理变量转化为客观的心身医学研究用诊断标准工具(见表1),进而被用于筛查、诊断心身疾病[4]。这种分类法的好处在于它摆脱了内科疾病的器质性和功能性二分法的束缚。

表 1　心身医学研究用诊断标准(1995 年版 DCPR)

健康焦虑(必须同时满足 A 和 B)

A. 对疾病的一般性担忧,关注疼痛和躯体先占观念(倾向于放大躯体感觉)持续时间少于 6 个月

B. 对合理医疗保证的焦虑可能迅速减轻,但新的焦虑依然有可能接踵而至

死亡恐惧(必须同时满足 A、B、C)

A. 有即将发生的死亡感和/或死亡信念冲击,即使这些恐惧没有客观的医学理由

B. 对于死亡相关信息(比如:葬礼、讣告)存在持续而显著的恐惧和回避行为;暴露于这些刺激会唤起直接的焦虑反应

C. 回避、焦虑预期和由此带来的苦恼明显影响了患者的功能水平

疾病恐惧(必须同时满足 A、B、C)

A. 没有理由地持续害怕遭遇一些特殊疾病(比如:艾滋病、癌症),尽管有合理的解释与保证,这种怀疑仍然不能消除

B. 这类恐惧与对慢性疾病的长期担忧不同(例如疑病症),患者的害怕通常集中在担心突然罹患某些疾病的可能性;惊恐发作可能是一种相关特征

C. 对于疾病的恐惧需不随时间改变,症状持续达到 6 个月

疾病否认(必须同时满足 A 和 B)

A. 存在疾病症状、体征和诊断,或需要治疗时,坚持否认自身患病,并且否认治疗的必要性(通常表现为:依从性差、对严重的持续的症状拖延就诊、反恐惧行为)。

B. 患者已经被提示过明确的疾病状况和自我管理方法

持续性躯体化(必须同时满足 A 和 B)

A. 功能性躯体障碍(如:纤维肌痛、疲劳、食管动力障碍、消化不良、肠易激综合征、神经循环无力、尿道综合征),持续时间超过 6 个月,造成患者极大困扰,导致重复医疗行为或造成生活质量下降

B. 其他器官系统自动唤醒症状(比如:心悸、出汗、震颤、脸红),夸大治疗的副反应,提示疼痛阈值低和高暗示性

转换性症状(必须同时满足 A、B、C)

A. 单独或多种影响运动、感觉功能的症状及损害,通常缺乏相应生理机制的解剖学证据,应有的体征或实验室检查结果亦常缺如,同时可能与临床特征不符;如果自动唤醒的症状(如:心悸、出汗、震颤、脸红)或功能性的医学障碍(纤维肌痛、疲劳、食管动力障碍、消化不良、肠易激综合征、神经循环无力、尿道综合征)存在,转换性症状应十分突出,造成患者苦恼,重复医疗行为,导致生活质量下降

B. 至少有以下 2 种特征存在:

　　1. 对症状的矛盾纠结(如:当他/她描述造成自己痛苦的症状时,却表现出轻松或不确定)

　　2. 戏剧性人格特征(富有色彩和戏剧性地表达,语言和外貌,极度依赖,高暗示性,情绪变化快)

　　3. 心理应激会使得症状成形,但患者没有意识到之间的联系

　　4. 患者曾经有过类似的症状,或者看到别人有过,寄希望于他人

C. 合理的医疗评估不能发现器质性病理证据来解释患者抱怨的躯体不适

继发于精神障碍的功能性躯体症状(必须同时满足 A、B、C)

A. 自动唤醒的症状(如:心悸、出汗、震颤、脸红)或功能性障碍(如:肠易激综合征、纤维肌痛、神经循环无力),造成患者苦恼,重复医疗行为,导致生活质量下降

B. 合理的医疗评估不能发现器质性病理证据来解释患者抱怨的躯体不适

C. 一种精神障碍(包括所涉及的临床表现中包含的躯体症状)发生在功能性躯体症状(如:疼痛障碍和心脏症状)之前

周年反应(必须同时满足 A、B、C)

A. 自动唤醒的症状(如:心悸、出汗、震颤、脸红)或功能性躯体障碍(如:肠易激综合征、纤维肌痛、神经循环无力)或转换性症状造成患者苦恼,重复医疗行为,导致生活质量下降

B. 合理的医疗评估不能发现器质性病理证据来解释患者抱怨的躯体不适

C. 通常发生于当患者到一定年龄,或发生在父母一方或亲近的家庭成员罹患疾病或者死亡的纪念日;患者自身没有意识到这之间的联系

沮丧(必须同时满足 A、B、C)

A. 患者意识到没能成功达成自己的期望(或他人的期望)或不能处理一些紧急的问题时产生的情感状态;患者感到无助、无望或准备放弃

B. 这种感觉状态广泛而持续(至少持续 1 个月)

C. 感觉几乎先于躯体疾病的临床症状发生或恶化疾病症状

易激惹(必须同时满足 A、B、C)

A. 一种在特殊环境下短时间发作的情感状态,但也可能广泛化慢性化;在这种状态下,患者或尝试加强控制情绪,或表现为愤怒言行的激烈爆发

B. 易激的经历对患者来说总是不愉快的,对怒气的合理排解通常表现为缺乏

C. 感觉引起应激相关的生理应答或加重疾病的症状

A 型行为(必须同时满足 A 和 B)

A. 9 项特征中至少具有 5 项:

　　1. 极端追求在期限内完成工作或其他活动

　　2. 时间紧迫感稳定和普遍

　　3. 表现出自动表达特征(快速和爆发性的说话,突然的身体移动,紧张的面部肌肉,手势)提示正处在时间造成的压力下

　　4. 敌意和愤世嫉俗

　　5. 易激情绪

　　6. 趋向于加快躯体活动

　　7. 趋向于加快精神活动

　　8. 极度渴望获得成就和认可

　　9. 高竞争性

B. 行为引起了应激相关的生理应答,从而加重了疾病的症状

述情障碍(满足 A)

A. 以下 6 个特征至少有 3 项存在:

　　1. 无法使用合理的语言描述情感

　　2. 趋向于描述细节而不是感觉(比如:事件发生的条件而不是感觉)

　　3. 生活中想象力贫乏

　　4. 思考的内容更多地关注与外部事件而不是想象或情绪

　　5. 没有意识到常见的躯体反应是与各种感觉联系在一起的

　　6. 偶发暴力行为,常见不恰当的情绪行为表达

　　自出版以来,DCPR 已被应用于多个国家的各种临床人群,包括功能胃肠功能紊乱[5]、心脏移植[6]、内分泌失调[7]以及癌症病人[8]等。它既能用来诊断"器质性"疾病,也能用于"功能性"疾病的评估[9],且此量表具有较好的可操作性和较高的可信区间(k:0.69～0.97)[10]。

　　国内李磊等[11]对原版 DCPR 进行翻译和校正并探讨中文版 DCPR 的临床价值,结果发现 95.4% 的抑郁和焦虑障碍患者存在至少一个 DCPR 症

状,接近 3/4 的患者至少存在两个 DCPR 症状,同时证实 DCPR 及多伦多述情障碍量表(TAS-20)诊断的述情障碍发生率无显著统计学差异。国外研究也证实,DCPR 和 TAS-20 具有良好的诊断一致性[5]。Guidi 等对 DCPR 及 DSM-5 相关诊断标准进行了比较,并认为相比于 DSM-5,DCPR 的敏感性及特异性均较高[12]。

三、2017 年版 DCPR

2017 年国际心身小组对 DCPR 的部分条目进行了修改,相比于 1995 年版 DCPR 更加关注异常行为与心理因素对健康的影响,新的版本增加了适应负荷、疑病症,并关注于压力(适应负荷)、个性(A 型行为、述情障碍)、患病行为(疑病症、疾病恐惧、死亡恐惧、健康焦虑、持续的躯体化、转换症状、周年反应、疾病否认)、心理表现(沮丧、易激惹、继发于精神障碍的功能性躯体症状)四大类共 14 个条目的内容,更加全面系统地对心身医学进行了诊断(见图 2)。

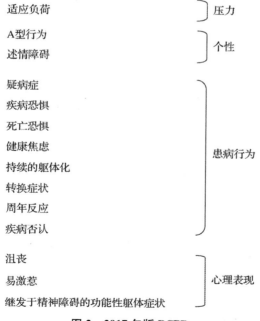

图 2　2017 年版 DCPR

相比于 1995 年版 DCPR,2017 年版新增以及改动的内容有:

(一) 新增的内容

1. 适应负荷

临床上我们常常能够观察到生活压力事件导致的健康损害,而数据采集的结构化分析方法的引入,又使内分泌系统、心血管系统、呼吸系统、胃肠道系统、自身免疫、皮肤和肿瘤疾病与早于其相关症状出现的生活事件的相关性得到证实[13]。事实上,在多因子的参照系中,生活压力事件可能会通过多种方式影响神经-内分泌免疫系统的调节功能[14]。当压力达到一定程度,则会引发由神经递质、促炎细胞因子和激素参与的反应[15]。这些反应可能在糖尿病、心血管疾病以及肿瘤等的发病机制中发挥着关键作用[16]。

McEwen[17] 基于稳态的定义即机体通过调节达到平衡稳定,明确了压力和其致病过程之间的关系。从这个角度出发,适应负荷反映的是日常生活中压力事件的累积效应。机体长期处于不断波动和升高的神经或神经内分泌反应,当这种反应超过个体应对能力的时候,适应负荷随即产生。

通常病人否认适应负荷是一种疾病症状的表现,因为他们并不知道症状的出现与压力积累之间的潜在联系。适应负荷与认知、生理功能和死亡率密切相关[17,18]。前额叶皮层、海马以及杏仁核是一些受影响最显著的脑区[19]。适应负荷可以通过特定的经过验证的临床度量标准进行评估[20]。这些标准在 DCPR 修订版中有所体现(见表 2)。

表 2　适应负荷(必须满足条件 A 和 B)

标准 A　近期存在以生活事件和/或者慢性压力形式出现的显著的疾病诱因;这种压力使个体负重或超过个体所能承受的范围
标准 B　压力源与以下 1~3 个症状相关,并且症状在压力源出现后的半年内现: 　(1) 至少存在下列两个症状:入睡困难、夜寐不安、早醒、精神不振、头昏眼花、广泛焦虑、易怒、悲伤、堕落 　(2) 严重影响其社会或职业功能 　(3) 严重影响其对外界事物的处理能力(对日常生活需求变得不知所措)

2. 疑病症

Mechanic 和 Volkart[21] 这样定义疾病行为——“不同的人对特定的症

状出现不同的感知、评价和行动(或不行动)方式"。随后,Mechanic[22]进行以下说明:"疾病行为涉及一系列个人对身体状况的反应,如何监控内部状态,定义和解释症状,归因,采取补救措施和利用各种正归和非正归的治疗行为。"

疾病行为是心身医学的一个核心特征,并且为那些无法进行传统分类的临床现象提供了一个很好的解释。疾病行为谱的临床表现包括很多症状,其中也包括 DSM-5 分类中省略的疑病症[23]。疑病症与疾病恐惧不同,表现为以下三点:① 疑病症只是表现出来持续的、长期的担忧,而疾病恐惧倾向于对自己的攻击[24];② 疑病症一般表现为寻求保证以及反复检查行为,而疾病恐惧往往会努力去避免与其疾病相关的内源性和外源性刺激[25];③ 疑病症的担忧不集中在某一特定的疾病,而疾病恐惧的担忧集中在某一个特定的疾病,并认为其不太可能转换为另一种疾病或另一系统的疾病[26]。

由于研究者们开发出了一种可以将疑虑这一疑病症核心症状很好逆转的心理治疗,且该种心理治疗在随机对照试验中已经通过验证[26],因此认为应该将疑病症保留(见表3)。

表 3　疑病症(必须满足标准条件 A~D)

标准 A　害怕或有担忧因躯体症状的误诊而致严重疾病
标准 B　经过反复的医学检查和保证、医生合理的讨论和解释,不能打消顾虑
标准 C　干扰持续的时间至少 6 个月
标准 D　这种关注导致明显的痛苦和/或社会和职业功能的损害

(二) 修改的内容

1. A 型行为和易激惹

人格特性的神经生理的表现为医疗机构预测疾病出现的症状和异常疾病行为提供了的病理生理学视角。潜在影响总体疾病的易损性的人格特性——A 型行为受到人们高度关注,但它与健康之间的关系仍然存在争议[27]。A 型行为来源于 1950 年代末在心脏病患者身上观察到的"情感-行为综合征",是由于个体的易患倾向和能察觉到的具体压力和挑战综合产生的[28]。其中发现具有 A 型行为的个体占存在患冠心病风险的受试者的36.1%,而仅占无心脏病受试人群的 10.8%[29]。A 型行为包括时间紧迫性、过度工作、敌意、快速的语言和行动竞争力及渴望成就,被描述为致力于用尽可能少的时间获得尽可能多的收益和积极参与长期不断的竞争。

而易怒可能是精神病综合征状的一部分,个人总是不愉快的,显著的临床表现为缺乏情绪的合理排解[30]。一些研究发现易激惹对疾病的发病过程以及不健康的生活方式的形成有着显著的影响[31]。应用 DCPR 的研究发现在医疗机构中具有心肌梗死、心脏移植、功能性胃肠道紊乱、癌症和皮肤病的患者,易激惹的患病率大约在 10%～15%[9],而内分泌疾病患者高达 46%[32]。

然而,1995 年版 A 型行为的诊断标准 B 以及易激惹的诊断标准 C 对两者的诊断限制过多,容易造成临床上的漏诊,且此标准条目的鉴定给临床医生带来极大的困难。为此,结合临床实际,2017 年版分别删除了 A 型行为的标准 B "行为引起了应激相关的生理应答,从而加重了疾病的症状"和易激惹的标准 C "感觉引起应激相关的生理应答或加重疾病的症状"这一条目。

2. 死亡恐惧

这组症状描述为死亡的恐怖感觉,在没有任何客观理由的情况下对将死的确信以及对于死亡有关消息的害怕,比如讣告通知。死亡恐怖症可能出现在惊恐障碍、疑病症和疾病恐怖症中以及其他心理症状中,具有较高的发病率[33]。

相比于 1995 年版 DCPR 有关死亡恐惧的诊断标准,2017 年版在其诊断标准 A 中加入了时间限制,即"在过去的六个月中,在没有实际危险,尽管有合理的评价,即使存在一些不良事件,医生也已经做过合理的处理,有合理的解释与保证的条件下,至少有两次出现有即将发生的死亡感和/或死亡信念冲击"。加入时间限制,使诊断标准更具严谨性,同时更好地指导临床医生对于死亡恐惧的诊断(见表 4)。

表 4　死亡恐惧(必须满足标准条件 A～C)

A. 在过去的六个月中,在没有实际危险,尽管有合理的评价,即使存在一些不良事件,医生也已经做过合理的处理,有合理的解释与保证的条件下,至少有两次出现有即将发生的死亡感和/或死亡信念冲击 B. 对于死亡相关信息(比如:葬礼、讣告)存在持续而显著的恐惧和回避行为;暴露于这些刺激会唤起直接的焦虑反应 C. 回避、焦虑预期和由此带来的苦恼明显影响了患者的功能水平

3. 转换症状

转换症状是根据 Engel 标准提出的,描述为感觉运动的缺失或者无法用器质性原因解释的随意运动,矛盾心理是其标准之一[33]。在一个以来自不同医疗机构的 1498 例患者为研究对象的实验中,利用 DCPR 诊断发现 4.5% 的受试者存在转换症状,而利用 DSM-IV 仅发现 0.4%[34]。

虽然 DCPR 在鉴定心身疾病比 DSM-IV 更具优势[3],但其关于转换症状的诊断顺序排列欠佳,对于此类患者的诊断应先排除器质性损害的可能。为此,2017 年版 DCRP 将其诊断标准 B 和诊断标准 C 的顺序做了对调(见表 5)。

表 5　转换症状(必须满足标准条件 A～C)

A. 单独或多种影响运动、感觉功能的症状及损害,通常缺乏相应生理机制的解剖学证据,应有的体征或实验室检查结果亦常缺如,同时可能与临床特征不符;如果自动唤醒的症状或持续的体征存在,转换性症状应十分突出,造成患者苦恼,重复医疗行为,导致生活质量下降 B. 合理的医疗评估不能发现器质性病理证据来解释患者抱怨的躯体不适 C. 下列四种特征至少有 2 项存在: 　1. 对症状的矛盾纠结(如:当他/她描述造成自己痛苦的症状时,却表现出轻松或不确定) 　2. 戏剧性人格特征(富有色彩和戏剧性地表达,语言和外貌,极度依赖,高暗示性,情绪变化快) 　3. 心理应激会使得症状成形,但患者没有意识到之间的联系 　4. 患者曾经有过类似的症状,或者看到别人有过,寄希望于他人

4. 沮丧

最早的 DCPR 中有关沮丧的定义是 Frank[35] 的沮丧综合征和 Schmale 以及恩格尔[36] 的欲放弃-放弃行为综合征的整合。研究表明沮丧在病患中具有较高的发生率[37]。

2017 年版 DCPR 沮丧诊断标准 A 和 C 变动较大,新的版本更显示它的两个不同的表述:无助(个人具有应对的能力,但缺乏足够的支持)和绝望(个体对于他/她独自面对的无法解决的问题时的一种感受)[38]。绝望和无助涉及 5-羟色胺能系统和去甲肾上腺素系统,而绝望很有可能与抑郁症更加相关,可能会为抑郁症严重程度的评估提供参考[39](见表 6)。

表 6 沮丧(必须满足标准条件 A 和 B,标准 C 是绝望特别说明)

A. 以感觉不能处理一些紧急的问题和/或缺乏他人足够的支持(无助)为特征;个人具有应对的能力
B. 这种感觉状态是长期的而广泛的(至少持续 1 个月)
C. 以坚信没有办法解决当前所遇到的问题和困难而有未能达到预期目标的挫败感为特征(无助)

四、中国版 DCPR

结合中国当前临床实际,袁勇贵等在 2017 版 DCPR 的基础上增加了神经质、体像障碍、逛医行为以及重大疾病/手术后的躯体不适共四个条目内容,并将疑病症改为疑病观念,关注于应激与个性(适应负荷、神经质、A 型行为、述情障碍)、患病行为(逛医行为、疑病观念、疾病恐惧、死亡恐惧、健康焦虑、持续的躯体化、转换症状、周年反应、疾病否认、体像障碍)、心理表现(沮丧、易激惹、重大疾病/手术后的躯体不适、继发于精神障碍的功能性躯体症状)三大方面共十八项内容,建立了符合中国国情的心身医学研究用诊断标准,即中国版心身医学研究用诊断标准(CDCPR)(见图 3):

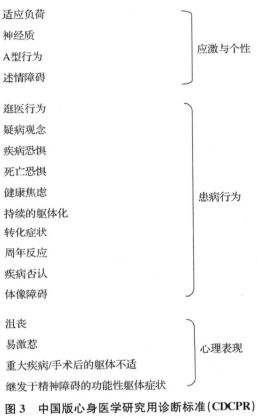

适应负荷	
神经质	
A型行为	应激与个性
述情障碍	

逛医行为	
疑病观念	
疾病恐惧	
死亡恐惧	
健康焦虑	患病行为
持续的躯体化	
转化症状	
周年反应	
疾病否认	
体像障碍	

沮丧	
易激惹	
重大疾病/手术后的躯体不适	心理表现
继发于精神障碍的功能性躯体症状	

图 3　中国版心身医学研究用诊断标准(CDCPR)

(一) 改变的内容

1. 疑病观念

对于健康,我们每个人都需要适度关注,但如果长期不切实际地高度关注,并且影响生活和工作,那演变成了疑病症。临床上,往往有些病人仅仅表现出过度关注自身健康。担心患上某种严重疾病,病程不超过 6 个月,也没有明显的社会功能损害,但却使病人处于紧张、焦虑和不安中,严重影响其自身健康。这种并未达到疑病症诊断标准的过度担忧的状态称为疑病观念[24](见表 7)。

表 7　疑病观念（必须满足标准条件 A~C）

标准 A	害怕或有担忧因躯体症状的误诊而致严重疾病
标准 B	经过反复的医学检查和保证，医生合理的讨论和解释不能打消顾虑
标准 C	这种关注导致明显的不良情绪和痛苦

（二）新增的内容

1. 神经质

神经质是一种稳定的人格特质，目前认为其主要表达两个方面的内容，即情绪稳定性和负性情绪倾向[40]。

情绪稳定-低神经质个体：常常表现为安静、轻松、自信、随和、稳重、自我克制；他们较少感受到大起大落的情绪体验，不易焦虑和沮丧不安。情绪不稳定-高神经质个体：常常喜怒无常、易兴奋激动紧张、多焦虑、郁闷、不安、敏感；他们在情绪上倾向于过度反应，在遭遇挫折或强烈的情绪体验时要经过长时间才能恢复常态[41]。

神经质是一种消极的人格特性，具有负性情绪倾向。神经质人格特征的个体对生活事件的应对能力较差，做事易冲动，同时会有更多的非理性观念，更容易遭受心理上的困扰。Wright 等[42]的研究发现对消极情感影响最大的人格因素是神经质因素。国内邱林等[43]在研究主观幸福感的结构及其与人格的关系中也发现个体的消极情感与神经质因素密切相关。过度神经质会增加患焦虑、抑郁障碍和其他情感障碍的风险。一项遗传学研究中发现神经质具有重性抑郁及广泛焦虑的基因易感性[44]。

而在大五人格因素模型中对于神经质的界定更为系统全面，在大五人格理论中，神经质又分为 6 个代表稳定的人格倾向子维度，每个子维度的差异都可能表现出不同的行为特征，可见神经质这种人格特性的复杂性。而神经质之所以与很多精神疾病都存在一定的关联，可能就是神经质的多子维度以及其自身的复杂性[45]。鉴于神经质特性与精神疾病的密切关系，因此中国版 DCPR 加入了这一人格因素的诊断（见表 8）。

表 8　神经质(满足标准 A)

标准 A　至少应该出现下列特征中的 5 条:
1. 常无缘无故感到无精打采和倦怠
2. 常常为自己不该做而做了的事、不该说而说了的话而紧张
3. 过分关注自身的不适或体验
4. 犹豫不决,常推迟或避免做出决定
5. 常常担心会发生可怕的事情
6. 对拒绝和批评过分敏感
7. 常为达不到自己的要求或目标而烦恼
8. 遇到一次难堪的经历后,会在一段很长的时间内还感到难受
9. 常忧心忡忡,有强烈的情绪反应

2. 逛医行为

逛医行为(Doctor shopping behaviors)是指病患为了更快更好地解决实际问题,而在医治过程中一再游走于不同医生及不同医院之间的行为表现。逛医行为的根源主要是患者对医生的不信任和对疾病的不了解,亦或是因为不愿意面对残酷的现实,通过不断地寻求医务服务而寻求任何一个可能的机会[46]。

这种现象存在以下几方面不利影响:① 对患者而言,由于反复游走于不同的医生和医院之间,造成每个医生都无法全面地对其病情进行掌握,最终患者得不到实质性的获利,往往是花费了大量的钱财而病情得不到改善,反而有时候还会加重;② 对医生而言,这种病人的存在无疑增加了其工作量,而反过来工作量的增加又降低了医生分配给每个人的看诊时间与看病质量,影响良好医患关系的建立;③ 就目前中国的就医环境而言,社会医疗负担在不断增大,而这种行为严重造成医疗资源的浪费,造成很多医疗资源不能得到有效利用,且逛医行为也有可能引起药物滥用。

为了更好地服务患者以及更好地利用医疗资源,需针对逛医行为进一步深入研究以及明确诊断(见表 9)。

表 9　逛医行为（必须满足标准条件 A～C）

标准 A	因害怕或担忧因躯体症状的误诊或误治而反复地要求医学检查和保证，或者反复游走于不同医生和不同医院之间
标准 B	这种行为持续的时间至少 6 个月
标准 C	这种行为导致明显的痛苦和/或社会和职业功能的损害

3. 体像障碍

体像障碍又称丑人综合征，是一种对轻微的或想象的外表缺陷的先占观念，这种观念垄断了患者的思想，患者常常不可忍受自身的"丑陋缺陷"，反复就诊和咨询医生，并由此产生心理痛苦的病症[47]。体像障碍具有较高的发病率，再加上此类患者还会出现较高的药物滥用史以及自杀倾向，因此需要引起社会的广泛重视[48]（见表 10）。

表 10　体像障碍（必须同时满足 A 和 B）

标准 A	近来关注外表上可见的、在别人看来不明显的或轻微的一个或多个缺陷（不足）
标准 B	为之烦恼，并表现出重复的行为（比如照镜子、过度修饰、抠挖皮肤及寻求保证）或精神活动（比如将自己的外貌和他人进行比较）

4. 重大疾病/手术后的躯体不适

临床上，在重大疾病或手术后患者往往会出现焦虑抑郁等情绪障碍，然而有相当一部分患者还甚至会出现头痛头晕、胸闷等功能性躯体不适症状，这些不适无法用疾病本身来解释，即使有些患者可能存在疾病本身所致的相关躯体症状，但其所主诉的躯体不适远远强于疾病本身引起的不适感[49]。这类患者往往被临床医师所忽视，从而严重影响患者疾病或术后恢复，导致其生存质量下降，我们将此类症状称之为重大疾病/手术后的躯体不适（见表 11）。

表 11　重大疾病/手术后的躯体不适（必须同时满足 A～C）

标准 A	发生于一种明确的重大躯体疾病（如心肌梗死）或手术后发生在功能性躯体症状
标准 B	合理的医疗评估不能发现器质性病理证据来解释患者抱怨的躯体不适
标准 C	功能性躯体不适症状，造成患者苦恼，重复医疗行为，导致生活质量下降

心身医学经历了两个世纪的发展壮大,已深入到综合医院的各个专业学科。而心身医学的研究领域仍处于起步阶段,心身疾病的流行病学调查、心身疾病的筛查工具的创制和诊疗规范制定以及心身疾病的疾病负担研究仍需进一步完善。

参考文献

[1] Lipowski ZJ. Psychosomatic medicine:past and present. Can J Psychiatry, 1986, 31(1):2 - 21.

[2] Wise TN. Psychosomatics:past, present and future. PsychotherPsychosom, 2014, 83(2): 65 - 69.

[3] Fava GA. Wise TN. Issues for DSM-V:psychological factors affecting either identified or feared medical conditions:a solution for somatoform disorders. Am J Psychiatry, 2007, 164(7):1002 - 1003.

[4] Mangelli L, Semprini F, Sirri L, et al. Use of the diagnostic Criteria for Psychosomatic Research (DCPR) in a community sample. Psychosomatics, 2006, 47(2): 143 - 146.

[5] Porcelli P, De Carne M. Criterion-related validity of the diagnostic criteria for psychosomatic research for alexithymia in patients with functional gastrointestinal disorders. PsychotherPsychosom, 2001, 70(4):184 - 188.

[6] Grandi S, Fabbri S, Tossani E, et al. Psychological evaluation after cardiac transplantation:the integration of different criteria. PsychotherPsychosom, 2001, 70 (4):176 - 183.

[7] Sonino N, Ruini C, Ottolini F, et al. Psychosocial correlates of endocrine disease. Eur Psychiatry, 2000, 15(suppl 2):345.

[8] Porcelli, P Rafanelli C. Criteria for psychosomatic research (DCPR) in the medical setting. Curr Psychiatry Rep, 2010, 12 (3): 246 - 254.

[9] Porcelli P, Guidi J. The clinical utility of the Diagnostic Criteria for Psychosomatic Research:a review of studies. PsychotherPsychosom, 2015, 84(5): 265 - 272.

[10] Galeazzi GM, Ferrari S, Mackinnon A, et al. Interrater reliability,prevalence,and

relation to ICD-10 diagnoses of the diagnostic Criteria for Psychosomatic Research in Consultation-Liaison psychiatric patients. Psychosomatics，2004，45（5）：386 - 339.

[11] 李磊，张钰群，杜向东，等. Fava 半定式访谈工具在中国抑郁和焦虑障碍患者中的运用. 中华行为医学与脑科学杂志，2016，25：16 - 20.

[12] Guidi J，Rafanelli C，Roncuzzi R，et al. Assessing psychological factors affecting medical conditions：comparison between different proposals. Gen Hosp Psychiatry，2013，35(2)：141 - 146.

[13] Theorell T. Evaluating life events and chronic stressors in relation to health. Adv Psychosom. Med，2012，32：58 - 71.

[14] Fink G. Stress Concept and Cognition，Emotion，and Behaviour. San Diego. 2016.

[15] Nemeroff CB. Paradise lost. the neurobiological and clinical consequences of child abuse and neglect. Neuron，2016，89(5)：892 - 909.

[16] Schöttker B，Saum KU，Jansen EH，et al. Associations of metabolic，inflammatory and oxidative stress markers with total morbidity and multi-morbidity in a large cohort of older German adults. Age Ageing，2016，45(1)：127 - 135.

[17] McEwen BS. Physiology and neurobiology of stress and adaptation：central role of the brain. Physiol Rev，2007，87(3)：873 - 904.

[18] McEwen BS，Bowles NP，Gray JD，et al. Mechanisms of stress in the brain. Nat Neurosci，2015，18：1353 - 1363.

[19] McEwen BS，Gianaros PJ. Stress-and allostasis-induced brain plasticity. Annu Rev Med，2011，62：431 - 445.

[20] Offidani E，Ruini C. Psychobiological correlates of allostatic overload in a healthy population. Brain BehavImmun，2012，26(2)：284 - 291.

[21] Mechanic D，Volkart EH. Illness behavior and medical diagnoses. J Health Hum Behav，1960，1：86 - 94.

[22] Mechanic D. Sociological dimensions of illness behavior. Soc Sci Med，1995，41(9)：1207 - 1216.

[23] American Psychiatric Association：Diagnostic and Statistical Manual of Mental

Disorders, ed 5. Washington, American Psychiatric Association. 2013.

[24] Fava GA, Grandi S. Differential diagnosis of hypochondriacal fears and beliefs. PsychotherPsychosom, 1991, 55(2-4):114-119.

[25] Noyes R, Carney CP, Langbehn DR. Specific phobia of illness: search for a new subtype. J Anxiety Disord, 2004, 18(4):531-545.

[26] Cosci F, Fava GA. The clinical inadequacy of the DSM-5 classification of somatic symptom and related disorders: an alternative trans-di-agnostic model. CNS Spectr, 2016, 21(4):310-317.

[27] Cosci F. Assessment of personality in psychosomatic medicine: current concepts. Adv Psychosom Med, 2012, 32: 133-159.

[28] Friedman M, Rosenman RH. Type A Behavior and Your Heart. New York, Knopf. 1974.

[29] Sirri L, Fava GA, Guidi J, et al. Type A behavior: a reappraisal of its characteristics in cardiovascular disease. Int J ClinPract, 2012, 66(9):854-861.

[30] Snaith RP, Taylor CM. Irritability. Br J Psychiatry, 1985, 147:127-136.

[31] Klabbers G, Bosma H, van den Akker M, et al. Cognitive hostility predicts all-cause mortality irrespective of behavioural risk at late middle and older age. Eur J Public Health, 2013, 23(4): 701-705.

[32] Sonino N, Navarrini C, Ruini C, et al. Persistent psychological distress in patients treated for endocrine disease. PsychotherPsychosom, 2004(2), 73:78-83.

[33] 吴爱勤. 心身医学分类诊断评估策略. 实用医院临床杂志, 2015, 12(06):1-6.

[34] Porcelli P, Fava GA, Rafanelli C, et al. Anniversary reactions in medical patients. J NervMent Dis, 2012, 200: 603-606.

[35] Frank JD. Persuasion and Healing. Baltimore, Johns Hopkins University Press, 1961.

[36] Schmale AH, Engel GL. The giving up-given up complex illustrated on film. Arch Gen Psychiatry, 1967, 17: 133-145.

[37] Tecuta L, Tomba E, Grandi S, et al. Demoralization: a systematic review on its clinical characterization. Psychol Med, 2015, 45(4): 673-691.

[38] Sweeney DR, Tinling DC, Schmale AH Jr. Differentiation of the 'giving-up' af-

fects-helplessness and hopelessness. Arch Gen Psychiatry, 1970, 23(4): 378 - 382.

[39] Benedetti F. The Patient's Brain. The Neuro-science behind the Doctor-Patient Relationship. Oxford, Oxford University Press, 2011.

[40] 李胜兰. 躯体疾病患者绝望水平及与神经质、领悟社会支持关系研究. 中南大学, 2014.

[41] Eysenck, H. J. Genetic and environmental contributions to individual differences: the three major dimensions of personality. J Pers, 1990, 52(1):81 - 90.

[42] Wright CI, Williams D, Feczko E, et al. Neuroanatomical correlates of extraversion and neuroticism. Cereb Cortex, 2006, 16(12):1809 - 1819.

[43] 邱林, 郑雪. 主观幸福感的结构及其与人格特质的关系. 应用心理学, 2005, (04): 330 - 335,353.

[44] Wadron JS, Malone SM, McGue M, et al. Genetic and environmental sources of covariation between early drinking and adult functioning. Psychol Addict Behav, 2017, 31(5):589 - 600.

[45] McCrae RR, Costa PT Jr. Validation of the five-factor model of personality across instruments and observers. J Pers Soc Psychol, 1987, 52(1):81 - 90.

[46] Sansone RA, Sansone LA. Doctor shopping: a phenomenon of many themes. InnovClinNeurosci, 2012, 9(11-12):42 - 46.

[47] Ahluwalia R, Bhatia NK, Kumar PS, et al. Body dysmorphic disorder: Diagnosis, clinical aspects and treatment strategies. Indian J Dent Res, 2017, 28(2):193 - 197.

[48] Kelly MM, Zhang J, Phillips KA. The prevalence of body dysmorphic disorder and its clinical correlates in a VA primary care behavioral health clinic. Psychiatry Res, 2015, 228(1):162 - 165.

[49] Ajiboye PO, Abiodun OA, Tunde-Ayinmode MF, et al. Psychiatric morbidity in stroke patients attending a neurology clinic in Nigeria. Afr Health Sci, 2013, 13 (3):624 - 631.

[作者:刘晓云　吴爱勤　袁勇贵]

附： Fava 半定式访谈工具在中国抑郁和焦虑障碍患者中的运用

摘　要

目的　应用 Fava 半定式访谈工具(DCPR)筛查中国抑郁和焦虑障碍人群中符合 DCPR 症状的发生率及其症状分布情况；并比较 A 型行为量表(TABP)、多伦多述情障碍量表(TAS-20)、简式健康焦虑量表(SHAI)与 DCPR 对相关症状的识别率是否存在差别。

方法　使用中文版 Fava 半定式访谈工具、17 项汉密尔顿抑郁量表(HAMD)及 14 项汉密尔顿焦虑量表(HAMA)对 110 例抑郁障碍患者和 41 名焦虑障碍患者进行评定，并与上述三个自评量表的症状发生率进行比较。

结果　151 例患者中，只有 7 例(4.6%)无 DCPR 症状，39 例(25.8%)存在 1 个 DCPR 症状者，存在 5 个以上 DCPR 症状者为 33 例(21.85%)。述情障碍[83 例(55.0%)]、沮丧[56 例(37.1%)]、A 型行为[53 例(35.1%)]和易激惹[37 例(24.5%)]最常见；抑郁和焦虑障碍患者只在周年反应的发生率上差异有统计学意义(16.4% 和 34.1%，$P<0.05$)。HAMA 与 DCPR 症状数量存在有统计学意义的相关性($r=0.167$；$P=0.041$)。DCPR 与 TAS-20 诊断的述情障碍发生率差异无统计学意义($\chi^2=2.069$，$P=0.150$)；DCPR 与 TABP 诊断的 A 型行为发生率差异有统计学意义($\chi^2=15.532$，$P=0.000$)；DCPR 与 SHAI 诊断的健康焦虑发生率差异有统计学意义($\chi^2=13.056$，$P=0.000$)。

结论　95.4% 的抑郁和焦虑障碍患者存在 1 个或 1 个以上 DCPR 症状，中文版 TAS-20 与 DCPR 对述情障碍的识别率无统计学意义的差别。

关键词　Fava 半定式访谈工具；抑郁障碍；焦虑障碍；述情障碍；A 型行为

针对躯体健康相关的心理因素的研究近 20 年来在中国得到了长足发展，特别述情障碍、A 型行为、易激惹及健康焦虑等越来越受到重视[1]。然而，各研究者采用不同的评估工具造成了研究结果同质性差以及不同研究者间交流障碍的问题；另一方面临床工作主要使用 DSM-Ⅳ、ICD-10 或 CCMD-3 等诊断分类体系，导致大量达不到诊断标准却存在社会心理易感因素或躯体化症状的患者未得到有效的关注。Fava 等[2]针对躯体健康相关心理状况筛查开发的半定式访谈工具(Fava's semi-structured diagnostic criteria for psychosomatic research，DCPR)将各种常见社会心理因素、异常疾病行为及躯体化症状转变为简单、可靠的半定式访谈工具。该访谈表弥补了传统精神障碍诊断标准的不足，具有较好的操作性，可用于躯体健康相关心理因素的筛查与诊断[3]。DCPR 已经在多个国家的综合及精神专科医院得到了应用[4]。国内尚缺乏类似的诊断工具。本研究首次调查了中文版 DCPR 症状在中国抑郁和焦虑障碍人群中的发生及分布情况，并分别比较 DCPR 诊断的述情障碍、A 型行为及健康焦虑与相关国内常用量表诊断的发生率。

一、对象与方法

(一) 对象

本研究在华东地区共 5 家医院(3 家精神病专科医院和 2 家综合医院)展开。入组标准：① 18～75 岁的住院患者；② 经精神科专科医生诊断符合 DSM-Ⅳ 抑郁障碍或焦虑障碍诊断标准；③ 汉族；④ 患者自愿参加本研究并签署知情同意。排除标准：① 患有或合并其他精神障碍患者；② 因躯体或精神状况无法进行有效访谈的患者。共有 151 例患者符合入组标准并完成评估，其中抑郁症 110 例、焦虑症 41 例，平均年龄(37.4±14.0)岁，其中男性 47 人(31.1%)、女性 104 人(68.9%)，已婚 114 人(75.5%)、未婚 37 (24.5%)。

(二) 方法

1. 评估流程

所有评估者均为临床研究经验的精神科或临床心理科专科医师(主治医师或以上)。根据入组及排除标准确定符合条件的患者，由评估者对患者进行访谈完成中文版 DCPR 半定式访谈表、17 项汉密尔顿抑郁量表(Hamilton depression scale, HAMD)及 14 项汉密尔顿焦虑量表(Hamilton anxiety scale, HAMA)。患者自行完成自评的病例报告表,包括自编的人口学资料调查表及多伦多述情障碍量表(Toronto alexithymia scale, TAS-20)、A 型行为量表(Type A behavior patern scale, TABP)及简式健康焦虑量表(Short health anxiety inventory, SHAI)等 3 份自评量表。若患者无法独立完成自评量表,由评估者大声朗读量表条目,再由患者考虑如何选择作答。项目实施前,所有评估者均进行了访谈和量表评估的一致性培训。

2. 评估工具

(1) DCPR:是 Fava[3] 领导的国际研究小组于 1995 年编制开发;经原作者同意,由东南大学附属中大医院心理精神科两名主治医师翻译成中文,经两名精神科主任医师校阅后,对译文做了进一步校正。该量表共包含 12 个症状,可分为三组:① 影响躯体健康的社会心理易感因素,包括述情障碍、A 型行为、易激惹和沮丧(demoralization);② 异常疾病行为,包括疾病恐惧、死亡恐惧、健康焦虑和疾病否认;③ 躯体化症状,包括继发于精神障碍的功能性躯体症状(Functional somatic symptoms secondary to psychiatric disorder, FSSSPD)、持续性躯体化、转换症状及周年反应。

(2) TAS-20:是 1994 年 Taylor 等在 TAS-26 的基础上修订而成,国内袁勇贵等[5] 将之翻译为中文并进行了信度与效度检验。

(3) TABP:是由中国心身医学协作组 1984 年制定,共有 60 题,包括时间匆忙感、争强好胜和谎分三个分量表[6]。

(4) SHAI:被认为是研究健康焦虑最有效的量表,其 18 个条目内部一致性高,对中国人群具有良好的信度与效度,≥15 分可认为存在健康焦虑[7]。

3. 统计

使用 SPSS 21.0 进行两样本 t 检验、卡方检验及 Pearson 相关分析,以 $P<0.05$ 为差异有统计学意义。

二、结果

(一) 抑郁和焦虑障碍患者的 DCPR 症状数量

在 151 例患者中,仅 7 例(4.6％)不符合任何 DCPR 的症状标准,144 例(95.4％)至少存在一个 DCPR 症状,其中存在 1 个 DCPR 症状者达 39 例(25.8％),存在 5 个以上 DCPR 症状者为 33 例(21.85％);抑郁和焦虑障碍患者的 DCPR 症状数量差异无统计学意义($\chi^2=1.247$,$P=0.536$)。见表 1。

表 1 抑郁和焦虑障碍患者 DCPR 症状数量比较 (个,％)

DCPR 症状数量(个)	例数 ($n=151$)	抑郁障碍 ($n=110$)	焦虑障碍 ($n=41$)	χ^2	P 值
0	7(4.6)	4(3.6)	3(7.3)	1.387	0.709
1	39(25.8)	30(27.3)	9(22.0)		
2～4	72(47.7)	53(48.2)	19(46.3)		
≥5	33(21.9)	23(20.9)	10(24.4)		

HAMD 评分与患者被诊断的 DCPR 症状数量的相关性无统计学意义($r=0.109$;$P=0.184$);而 HAMA 评分与患者被诊断的 DCPR 症状数量存在相关性,有统计学意义($r=0.167$;$P=0.041$),见图 1。

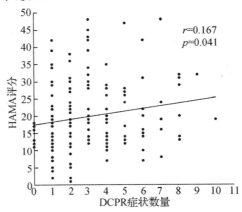

图 1 DCPR 症状数量与 HAMA 评分的相关性

（二）各 DCPR 症状的发生率

最常见的 DCPR 症状与社会心理易感因素有关：述情障碍 83 例（55.0%）、沮丧 56 例（37.1%）、A 型行为 53 例（35.1%）和易激惹 37 例（24.5%）。较少见的症状为转换症状 13 例（8.6%），疾病恐惧 18 例（11.9%），健康焦虑 29 例（19.2%）及死亡恐惧 29 例（19.2%）。本研究进一步比较了各症状在抑郁和焦虑障碍患者的发生率间是否存在差异。在周年反应的发生率上，抑郁障碍患者（16.4%）低于焦虑障碍患者（34.1%），差异有统计学意义（$\chi^2 = 5.655$，$P < 0.05$）；在其他 DCPR 症状的发生率上抑郁和焦虑障碍患者差异无统计学意义。见表 2。

表 2　焦虑及抑郁障碍患者各 DCPR 症状发生率比较　　　　　（例，%）

DCPR 症状	例数（$n=151$，%）	排序	抑郁障碍（$n=110$，%）	焦虑障碍（$n=41$，%）	χ^2	P 值
健康焦虑	29(19.2)	9	18(16.4)	11(26.8)	2.108	0.147
疾病恐惧	18(11.9)	11	10(9.1)	8(19.5)	2.177	0.140
死亡恐惧	29(19.2)	9	20(18.2)	9(22.0)	0.273	0.601
疾病否认	35(23.2)	5	24(21.8)	11(26.8)	0.421	0.516
FSSSPD	33(21.9)	7	23(20.9)	10(24.4)	0.212	0.645
持续躯体化	35(23.2)	5	24(21.8)	11(26.8)	0.421	0.516
转换症状	13(8.6)	12	9(8.2)	4(9.8)	0.000	1.000
周年反应	32(21.2)	8	18(16.4)	14(34.1)	5.655	0.017
A 型行为	53(35.1)	3	37(33.6)	16(39.0)	0.381	0.537
易激惹	37(24.5)	4	29(26.4)	8(19.5)	0.758	0.384
沮丧	56(37.1)	2	44(40.0)	12(29.3)	1.474	0.225
述情障碍	83(55.0)	1	60(54.5)	23(56.1)	0.029	0.865

（三）DCPR 与 TAS-20、TABP、SHAI 症状诊断率对比

述情障碍的发生率 DCPR 为 55.0%，而使用 TAS-20 评定为 36.4%，差异无统计学意义（$\chi^2 = 2.069$，$P = 0.150$）；A 型行为的发生率 DCPR 为

35.1%,而使用 TABP 评定为 44.4%,差异具有统计学意义($\chi^2=15.532$, $P=0.000$);健康焦虑的发生率 DCPR 为 19.2%,而使用 SHAI 评定为 56.3%,差异有统计学意义($\chi^2=13.056$,$P=0.000$)。

三、讨论

本研究纳入了来自华东地区的五家医院的 151 例抑郁和焦虑障碍患者,结果表明我国抑郁和焦虑障碍患者中 DCPR 症状的发生率高(95.4%的患者存在至少一个或更多 DCPR 症状),其中将近 3/4 的患者同时存在两个或以上症状。据我们所知,这是首个将 DCPR 用于在中国人群筛查躯体健康相关心理因素的研究。

本研究发现各 DCPR 症状中,50.6%与社会心理易感因素有关,主要包括了述情障碍、沮丧、A 型行为和易激惹。识别影响躯体状况的社会心理易感因素一直是临床研究者关注的重点内容。DSM-IV 描述了影响躯体状况的心理因素(Psychological Factors affecting Medical Conditions,PFAMC)的分类及诊断标准,然而由于标准的模糊性,该诊断条目对当前临床实践几乎无实质性帮助[8]。DSM-5 将 PFAMC 的相关诊断条目归入躯体症状及相关障碍类目中。Guidi 等[9]比较了 DCPR 及 DSM-5 标准后认为 DCPR 的敏感性及特异性均优于 DSM-5。DCPR 症状数量与抑郁严重程度相关性无统计学意义,尽管其与焦虑严重程度存在有统计学意义的正相关,但相关程度极低($r=0.167$),DCPR 症状独立于焦虑及抑郁症状之外。

述情障碍是一种难以准确识别和表达情感的人格特质,与焦虑及抑郁关系密切,且显著增加各种躯体健康问题的风险[10-11]。国内使用 TAS-20 发现抑郁障碍患者中述情障碍的发生率为 43%[12],且述情障碍能够增加有述情障碍抑郁症患者的过度概括化自传体记忆的严重程度[13],并增加神经质人格对抑郁的预测能力[14]。理论上,DCPR 述情障碍诊断标准的部分条目分别对应了 TAS-20 的三个因子,即难以识别自己的情感、难以描述自己的情感及外向性思维。本研究在抑郁和焦虑障碍患者中分别使用 DCPR 及

TAS-20 诊断的述情障碍发生率差异无统计学意义。国外研究也证实，DCPR 和 TAS-20 有着良好的诊断一致性[15]。

沮丧是一种"正在放弃-已经放弃"复合体（givingup-givenup complex），它主要包括无助感、绝望感和无意义感[16]。沮丧在本研究中的发生率为 37.1%。沮丧可能是抑郁障碍发生的先兆症状[17]，然而，沮丧并不等同于抑郁，它是一种独立的临床症状，且发生率高于抑郁障碍[16]。有学者将 DCPR 的沮丧症状与轻微的抑郁[18]或恶劣心境[19]相混淆，如何恰当地区分这些概念，还有待进一步研究揭示。

A 型行为与易激惹在本研究中发生率也较高。DCRP 诊断的 A 型行为与易激惹存在相关[20]，易激惹可能是 A 型行为的一部分[2]。TABP 诊断的 A 型行为者容易出现焦虑、厌烦及失望等负面情绪[21]。一般认为 A 型行为与焦虑的关系较抑郁更密切，使用 TABP 评估发现，焦虑障碍患者中 A 型行为发生率是抑郁障碍的两倍[22]，而本研究的焦虑障碍与抑郁障碍患者 A 型行为发生率无差异，结果的不一致可能与使用不同的评估工具有关。本研究中 DCPR 与 TABP 诊断的 A 型行为的发生率差异有统计学意义，TABP 将时间紧迫感和争强好胜描述为 A 型行为的两个主要特征，而 DCPR 在此之外，还强调了"行为引起了应激相关的生理应答（如心悸、出汗或呼吸急促等），从而加重了疾病的症状"。

DCPR 的周年反应是指患者在家庭成员患重病或死亡的年龄或纪念日出现的一系列功能性躯体症状，如自动唤醒的症状、功能性躯体障碍或转换性症状[2]。本研究发现，周年反应的发生率在抑郁和焦虑障碍患者中差异有统计学意义（分别 34.1% 和 16.1%）。国外一项针对综合医疗机构患者的研究发现，DCPR 诊断的周年反应患者中焦虑障碍和心境障碍的共病率分别为 27.8% 和 20.4%[23]。心悸、出汗、震颤和脸红等自动唤醒症状并不能完全与焦虑的躯体症状相区分，这也许是周年反应与焦虑障碍共病率高的原因之一。

尽管本研究中抑郁和焦虑障碍患者健康焦虑的发生率（19.2%）相对较

低,但仍远高于健康人群约 5％的发生率[24],抑郁和焦虑症状与健康焦虑的关系密切[25]。DCPR 与 SHAI 在健康焦虑的诊断一致性差,两量表的差异值得进一步研究。

总之,DCPR 具有重要的临床价值,本研究中 95.4％的抑郁和焦虑障碍患者存在 1 个或以上 DCPR 症状,影响躯体状况的社会心理易感因素最常见,中文版 DCPR 与 TAS-20 对述情障碍的识别率无显著差别。

参考文献

[1] Yuan Y,Wu A,Jiang. W Psychosomatic medicine in China [J]. Psychother Psychosom, 2015, 4 (1)：59 - 60.

[2] Fava GA,Freyberger HJ,Bech P,et al. Diagnostic criteria for use in psychosomatic research [J]. Psychother Psychosom,1995,63 (1):1 - 8.

[3] Fava GA,Sonino N,Wise TN. Principles of psychosomatic assessment[J]. Adv Psychosom Med,2012,32:1 - 18.

[4] Porcelli P,Guidi J. The Clinical Utility of the Diagnostic Criteria for Psychosomatic Research:A Review of Studies[J]. Psychother Psychosom,2015,84(5):265 - 272.

[5] 袁勇贵,沈鑫华,张向荣,等. 多伦多述情障碍量表(TAS-20)的信度和效度研究[J]. 四川精神卫生,2003,16(1):25 - 27.

[6] 张作记. 行为医学量表手册[M/ CD]. 2005,北京:中华医学电子音像出版社. 157 - 186.

[7] Zhang Y,Liu R,Li G,et al. The reliability and validity of a Chinese-version Short Health Anxiety Inventory:an investigation of university students [J]. Neuropsychiatr Dis Treat,2015,11:1739 - 1747.

[8] Fava GA,Wise TN. Issues for DSM-V:psychological factors affecting either identified or feared medical conditions:a solution for somatoform disorders[J]. Am J Psychiatry,2007,164(7):1002 - 1003.

[9] Guidi J,Rafanelli C,Roncuzzi R,et al. Assessing psychological factors affecting medical conditions:comparison between different proposals[J]. Gen Hosp Psychiatry,2013,35(2):141 - 146.

[10] 卢妍妍,阎琳,蒋珊,等. 伴躯体症状抑郁症患者皮质醇与述情障碍的相关性 [J]. 中华行为医学与脑科学杂志,2014,23(6):511-513.

[11] 唐秋萍,张玉桃,朱熊兆. 述情障碍对抑郁症状的影响 [J]. 中华行为医学与脑科学杂志,2011,20(6):545-546.
Tang QP,Zhang YT,Zhu XZ,et al. The Effect of Alexithymia on depression [J]. Chin J Behav Med Brain Sci,2011,20(6):545-546.

[12] 张金香,杨秋兰. 抑郁症患者的述情障碍与焦虑、抑郁的相关性研究 [J]. 中国健康心理学杂志,2007,15(6):493-494.

[13] 柳艳松,王军,孙玉军,等. 有述情障碍与无述情障碍抑郁症患者自传体记忆比较 [J]. 中华行为医学与脑科学杂志,2015,24(9):808-811.

[14] 张玉桃,吴岚,张生丛,等. 抑郁相关人格维度与人格特质的关系及其对抑郁的影响 [J]. 中华行为医学与脑科学杂志,2014,23(7):615-618.

[15] Porcelli P,De Carne M. Criterion-related validity of the diagnostic criteria for psychosomatic research for alexithymia in patients with functional gastrointestinal disorders[J]. Psychother Psychosom, 2001,70(4):184-188.

[16] Tecuta L,Tomba E,Grandi S,et al. Demoralization:a systematic review on its clinical characterization[J]. Psychol Med,2015,45(4):673-691.

[17] Rickelman BL. Demoralization as a Precursor to Serious Depression [J]. Journal of the American Psychiatric Nurses Association,2002,8(1):9-19.

[18] Rafanelli C,Offidani E,Gostoli S,et al. Psychological correlates in patients with different levels of hypertension[J]. Psychiatry Res, 2012,198(1):154-160.

[19] Rafanelli C,Milaneschi Y,Roncuzzi R,et al. Dysthymia before myocardial infarction as a cardiac risk factor at 2.5-year follow-up[J]. Psychosomatics,2010,51(1):8-13.

[20] Sirri L,Fava GA,Guidi J,et al. Type A behaviour:a reappraisal of its characteristics in cardiovascular disease[J]. Int J Clin Pract, 2012,66(9):854-861.

[21] 马惠霞,苏世将,聂胜昀. 大学生 A 型行为类型及其学业情绪特点 [J]. 心理与行为研究,2009(03):193-197.

[22] 郭苏皖,隋毓秀,张向荣,等. 焦虑症与抑郁症的 A 型行为比较[J]. 四川精神卫生,2002,15(2):70-71.

［23］ Porcelli P,Fava GA,Rafanelli C,et al. Anniversary reactions in medical patients
[J]. J Nerv Ment Dis,2012,200(7):603-606.

［24］ Sunderland M,Newby JM,Andrews G. Health anxiety in Australia：prevalence,
comorbidity,disability and service use[J]. Br J Psy chiatry,2013,202(1):56-61.

［25］ Bourgault-Fagnou MD, Hadjistavropoulos HD. Understanding health anxiety a-
mong community dwelling seniors with varying degrees of frailty[J]. Aging Ment
Health,2009,13(2):226-237.

［作者及发表刊物：

李磊,张钰群,杜向东,沈鑫华,杨忠,石元洪,刘瑞,王桥,吴爱勤,袁勇贵.
Fava半定式访谈工具在中国抑郁和焦虑障碍患者中的应用[J].中华行为
医学与脑科学杂志,2016,25(9):807-811.］

新评估

Reliability and validity of a new post-stroke depression scale in Chinese population

Background: Nowadays there is still a lack of effective method to e-valuate post-stroke depression. To distinguish patients with and without depression after stroke reliably, this study proposes a new PostStroke Depression Scale (PSDS).

Methods: PSDS was developed based on various depression scales and clinician experiences. 158 stroke patients who were able to fin-ish PSDS and Hamilton Depression Rating Scale (HDRS) were re-cruited. Cronbach α, Spearman rank coefficient and Kruskal – Wal-lis test were respectively used to examine reliability, internal con-sistency and discriminate validity. Then the Receiver Operating Characteristic (ROC) curve was used to determine the ability of scale and categorized scales to the range of depression. Finally, the factors of the PSDS were classified by average clustering analysis.

Results: The Cronbach α of PSDS was 0.797 (95% CI) indicted a good reliability. The Spearman correlation coefficient between PSDS and HDRS was 0.822 ($P < 0.001$) showed an excellent congruent validity. The discriminate validity displayed significant difference between patients with and without depression ($P < 0.001$). 6/24 was set to be the cut-off value by ROC analysis. Moreover, the different severity was distin-guished by the value 6/24, 15/24 and 17/24.

Limitations: The small sample size maybe the main limitation, the larger sample used in different fields according sex, age and side-le-sion was needed to verity the results. The cut off value calculated by ROC curve maybe react the severity of the disease to some ex-tent, but it is not absolute.

Conclusions: PSDS is a valid, reliable and specific tool for evaluating post-stroke depression patients and can be conveniently utilized.

Key words：stroke；Depression；Assessment；Post-Stroke Depression Scale(PSDS)

中 文 摘 要

卒中后抑郁评估量表在中国人群中的信效度研究

岳莹莹　刘　瑞　陆　建　王晓菁
张石宁　吴爱勤　王　桥　袁勇贵

目的：当前对于卒中后抑郁(post stroke depression，PSD)患者，仍缺乏有效的评估量表进行早期筛查，为了能够有效识别 PSD 患者，我们制定了一个新的卒中后抑郁评估量表(post stroke depression scale，PSDS)。

方法：该量表根据已有的抑郁评估量表和临床医生经验制定。本研究入组 158 例脑卒中患者，采用汉密尔顿抑郁量表(Hamilton Depression Rating Scale，HDRS)和 PSDS 对抑郁症状进行评估，通过 Cronbach α 系数、Spearman 秩相关、Kruskal-Wallis 检验对该量表的信度、内部一致性和区分效度进行检测；之后通过受试者工作特征曲线(receiver operating characteristic，ROC)和约登指数(Youden index，YI)对量表的有效性进行测定和界值划分；最后通过聚类分析方法寻找 PSD 的特异症状。

结果：PSDS 的 Cronbach α 为 0.797，表明该量表有较好的信度。PSDS 和 HDRS 的相关系数为 0.822($P<0.001$)，PSD 和卒中非抑郁(Non-PSD)患者的 PSD-S 评分存在显著差异($P<0.001$)表示其有较好的聚合效度和区分效度。ROC 曲线和 YI 指数示 6/24，15/24，分别为可疑/轻度抑郁，中重度抑郁的界值。

局限：本研究样本量较小，未来可以在大样本中通过对年龄、性别和卒中部位进行分层研究，界值划分在一定程度上反应了抑郁严重程度。

结论：PSDS 是简单易行的自评量表，在卒中人群中具有较好的信度和效度，可以用来对卒中幸存者进行广泛筛查，实现 PSD 的早期发现。

关键词：卒中；抑郁；评估；卒中后抑郁评估量表

1 Introduction

Post-stroke depression is a frequent complication that worsens rehabilitation outcomes, quality of life and confers substantial risk for suicide (de Man-van Ginkel et al., 2012; Pompili et al., 2012). A pooled estimate indicates that depressive symptoms are present in one third of all stroke survivors at any time during the follow-up (de Man-van Ginkel et al., 2013; Zhang et al., 2012). Increasing evidence shows that regularly antidepressant treatment will lead to decreased depression symptoms and improved functional status (Loubinoux et al., 2012). Therefore, the early detection of poststroke depression is essential to optimize the recovery of stroke patients and avoid unfortunate incidents.

The diagnosis criteria of post-stroke depression are virtually unclear because there is no accurate description of this disease in the three international diagnosis systems, including Diagnostic and Statistical Manual of Mental Disorder, Fourth Edition (DSM-IV) by American Psychiatry Association, the International Classification of Disease, Tenth Edition of the World Health Organization and Chinese Classification of Mental Disorders, Third Version. Among them, DSM-IV is one of the most common diagnostic criteria at present (Kang et al., 2013), but it just recommends that post-stroke depression is distinguished from a "Mood Disorder due to a General Medical Condition" (§293.83) when the mood disturbance is judged to be a direct consequence of a medical condition such as stroke. It was described as "depressive disorder due to another medical condition" in the DSM-5 published in May, 2013. The etiology is nearly unknown and confused by many factors, so the diagnostic nosology is focused on clinical manifestations, duration of disorders and interference with social function.

The evaluation of depression in the stroke patients is performed generally using the scales developed for the psychiatric population (Gabaldon et al., 2007), which include the Hamilton Depression Rating Scale (HDRS) (Hamilton, 1960), Beck Depression Inventory (Beck et al., 1961), Montgomery Asberg Depression Rating Scale (Montgomery and Asberg, 1979), Zung Self-rating Depression Scale (Zung, 1965) and Geriatric Depression Screening Scale (Yesavage et al., 1983). HDRS has been one of the most widely used in the study of post-stroke depression and has been shown to be a reliable instrument (Bjerg et al., 1997; Aben et al., 2001; Aben et al., 2002). Originally, it consists of 17 items that evaluate the symptoms of depression, in which 3 items are sleep-related. However, there have been some concerns raised about their low specificity (Salter et al., 2007). For example, the use of verbal skills to diagnose and measure depression is a matter for debate since there is no instrument designed specifically for patients who have suffered from stroke that usually caused physical and cognitive impairments (Kang et al., 2013). On the other hand, a state of agitation or psychomotor retardation, insomnia, or significant loss of weight that may be directly related to the somatic disorder accounted for a large part percentage of the total score biased to depression. Furthermore, motor aphasia patients may even make it difficult to communicate with patients. Several scales have been proposed for specifically evaluation for aphasic patients, including the Visual Analog Mood Scales (Arruda et al., 1999), Stroke Aphasic Depression Questionnaire (Lincoln et al., 2000) and the Aphasic Depression Rating Scale (Benaim et al., 2004). However Stroke Aphasic Depression Questionnaire is commonly used by caregiver or rehabilitators through the observation of the patients, but few study has been used by nurses' or rehabilitation observation and proxy ratings in assessing depression after stroke patients. Then a test named post-stroke depression rating scale specifically devised for post-stroke patients was consisted of 10 sections including catastrophic reaction as well as difficulty in emotional control and each section has different subtype (Gainotti et al., 1997). Maybe some items that have not been commonly accepted limit their wide-spread application by clinical and scientific research of post-stroke depression patients (Colasanti et al., 2010; Spalletta and Robinson, 2010).

Because of no specific self-rating assessment of post-stroke depression patients, this study is aimed to develop a new PostStroke Depression Scale (PSDS) in Chinese population and then verify the reliability and validity of the scale.

2 Materials and methods

2.1 The development of the PSDS

The selection of items was as followed: first, 55 items were collected after being analyzed, arranged and merged from HDRS, Zung Self-rating Depression Scale, Beck Depression Inventory, Montgomery Asberg Depression Rating Scale, Aphasic Depression Rating Scale, Stroke Aphasic Depression Questionnaire, Visual Analog Mood Scales, Post-Stroke Depression Rating Scale, Center for Epidemiologic Studies Depression Scale (Radloff, 1977), the Hospital Anxiety and Depression Scale (Zigmond and Snaith, 1983) and the Patient Health Questionnaire Depression Scale-9 (Williams et al., 2005). Second, 17 items were selected by 10 senior psychiatrists or neurologists according to their clinical experiences in our research group. Then, these items were emailed to the national experts to choose the common symptoms in depressive patients after stroke according to their clinical experiences. Replies were received from 65 chief doctors consisting of 39 psychiatrists and 26 neurologists. The PSDS consisted of 8 items [decreased speech (do not want to speak), easy fatigability, easy to cry, insomnia (waking up too early), feeling of decreased capability, suicidal ideation, feeling of difficult to recover, more irritable than usual] which were most selected by more than half – experts after statistics (see Supplementary material). PSDS is a self – rating scale, the subjects were asked to read each of the 8 items and carefully decided how often the statement describes according their feeling during the last 7 days in the following four quantitative terms: absent, some of the time, part of the time, or most of the time. A value of 0, 1, 2, and 3 is assigned to a response depending upon whether the item was positive or negative. The PSDS is constructed so that the more depressed subjects and his complaint will have a higher score on the scale. Add up the score of each item for a total score and the highest possible score is 24.

2.2　Participant selection

This study was approved by the Medical Ethics Committee for Clinical Research of Zhongda Hospital Affiliated to Southeast University. A prospective study was conducted in 2 cooperation hospitals: Nanjing Ruihaibo Rehabilitation Hospital and Nanjing Brain Hospital in 2013. A total of 158 patients were recruited and they were all given written informed consent. To be enrolled in our study, participants are required to meet the following criteria: (1) all participants with ischemic stroke and intracerebral hemorrhage determined by Computed Tomography (CT) or Magnetic Resonance Imaging (MRI) data; (2) each participant evaluated HDRS and PSDS; (3) participants were antidepressant-naïve, and the age of onset was under 80 years; (4) participants were free of other major psychiatric disorders, including schizophrenia, bipolar disorder, substance abuse (caffeine, nicotine and alcohol) (American Psychiatric Association, 1994), neurodegenerative illness, severe physical illnesses and other medical illnesses; (5) participants were free of anosognosia, neglect, hemianopia, cortical blindness, amnesia, aphasia, dementia and other symptoms hindered assessment.

Diagnostic evaluations of post-stroke depression were carefully conducted on all participants who fulfilled the following diagnostic criteria combined with the previous literature by two trained senior psychiatrists. Five aspects were included in the diagnostic criteria: (1) had stroke before, or stroke occurs earlier than depressive symptoms; (2) met at least two depressive symptoms except core criterion symptoms of depressed mood and loss of interest or pleasure in nine symptoms of major depressive disorder in DSM-IV; (3) impairment to fit personal and work functioning (not induced by somatic disorder), the motor deficits since stroke were evaluated by Barth Index (Mahoney and Barthel, 1965); (4) depressive symptoms lasting more than 1 week; (5) free of other major psychiatric disorders, including schizophrenia, bipolar disorder, substance abuse (caffeine, nicotine and alcohol) (see Supplementary material).

2.3 Data analysis

SPSS 18.0 software (SPSS, Inc, Chicago, IL) was used to calculate the reliability and validity of PSDS and MATLAB (R 2012b) was to clustering analysis and multiple linear regression. We would illustrate the PSDS from the following five aspects.

First, in order to ensure reliability of the results, PASS 13 was used to calculate the power while α was set to 0.05.

Second, the reliability of PSDS and HDRS was assessed by Cronbach α which evaluated the internal consistency of each items. In the exploratory analysis, the value of Cronbach α 0.6—0.9 indicates good consistency reliability (Duncan et al. , 1999).

Third, the validity of PSDS was assessed by Spearman rank correlation coefficient and Kruskal – Wallis test (Rosner, 2004). Validity is used to show the accuracy, usefulness of assessment which included criterion validity, content validity and construct validity. Content validity contains congruent validity and discriminated validity. The congruent validity was calculated by the Spearman rank correlation coefficient and discriminate validity was estimated by Kruskal – Wallis test. In order to assess the criterion validity of PSDS, Spearman rank correlation coefficient was used to indicate the relationship between each item and the total score. A high correlation during -1 to -0.5 and 0.5 to 1 indicates good consistency and shows that PSDS could be used to evaluate the depression (McCrate et al. , 2011). The items which Spearman rank correlation coefficients were larger than 0.6 were considered to be the specific characteristics of post-stroke depression patients. In order to test whether the suspected specific characteristics can explain the depression, the correlation between the total score of four suspected characteristics of post-stroke depression and HDRS total score was calculated.

Fourth, the diagnose cut-off score was developed by Youden Index combing sensitivity value and specificity value (Fluss et al. , 2005), which resulted from ROC curve. The areas of ROC curve were rational index of the whole diagnostic precision of the test. Youden Index was calculated by the formula:

$$\text{Youden Index} = \text{sensitive value} + \text{specificity value} - 1 \qquad (1)$$

The maximum of Youden Index is the best cut-off score. To verify the accuracy and effectivity of this cut-off value, we calculated the accordance rate compared with HDRS and used multiple linear regression to observe the comparison directly.

Finally, the main factors of the PSDS were classified by an average clustering analysis method.

3 Results

From all participating patients, data were collected regarding potential risk factors for post-stroke depression (Hackett and Anderson, 2005). These included socio-demographic and strokerelated factors medical history concerning vascular risk factors and vascular diseases (van Swieten et al. , 1988). Details are described in Table 1. Table 2 describes the relative stage of stroke patients. For a variable to be considered candidate predictor of post-stroke depression, it had to be easily collected in a clinical setting with a view to future applicability. Consequently, the data collected were a proportion of the data normally collected in hospital care.

There were 101 stroke patients without depression (63. 92%) and 57 post-stroke depression patients (36. 08%) which contained 43 males and 14 females in this study.

Table 1　Characteristics of study sample

Patients	Post-stroke depression patients ($n=57$)	Patients without depression ($n=101$)
Sex ($n\%$)		
Male	43(75. 44)	71(70. 3)
Female	14(24. 56)	30(29. 7)
Age (y)		
Mean (SD; min-max)	64. 4(11. 2; 32—92)	61. 1(10. 5; 32—83)
Marital status ($n\%$)		
Single	0(0)	1(0. 99)
Married/cohabiting	51(89. 47)	94(93. 07)

Widowed/divorced	6(10. 5)	6(5. 94)
Type of stroke ($n\%$)		
Intracerebral hemorrhage	13(22. 8)	35(34. 65)
Ischemic stroke	45(78. 94)	67(66. 34)
Vascular risk actors($n\%$)		
Diabetes mellitus	14(24. 56)	30(29. 7)
Hypertension	48(84. 21)	81(80. 2)
Dyslipidemia	6(10. 53)	8(7. 92)
Impaired renal function	3(5. 26)	3(2. 97)
Smoking	20(35. 09)	45(44. 55)
Alcohol consumption	16(28. 07)	30(29. 7)

Table 2　The duration distribution of the study sample.

Duration distribution	Stage	The number of patients
7 days	Acute	4
7 days – 1 month	Subacute	3
1 mouth – 1 year		55
1 year – 10 years	Chronic	77
More than 10 years		19

3. 1　Power of test

β is the probability of accepting a false null hypothesis which should be small when α is 0. 05. Conventionally a test with a power greater than 0. 8 (or $\beta \leqslant 0.2$) is considered statistically powerful (Park, 2008). Through the analysis of PASS 13, when the size of sample is 130, β is 0. 118, so its power is 88%. If the size of sample is 170, β is 0. 05, so its power is 95%. In this study, the size is 158, so the power between 88% and 95%. The value of power is enough to show patients with and without depression had significant difference and this study is effective.

3.2　Reliability

Cronbach α was used to estimate the reliability of scales. The Cronbach α of PSDS and HDRS is 0.797 (95% CI) and 0.643 (95% CI) respectively, which shows that PSDS has a better reliability than HDRS.

3.3　Validity

All data of subjects were used to calculate the Spearman rank correlation of PSDS and HDRS scores. The correlation coefficient was 0.822 ($P <$ 0.001) which showed a good congruent validity. In hence it can be used to evaluate depression. Then, we used Kruskal - Wallis Test to calculate the discriminate validity of PSDS and the result showed PSDS had significant difference between patients with and without depression after stroke. The result demonstrated a significant effect on estimating depression in stroke patients ($P < 0.001$). The boxes plot of the group of poststroke patients and stroke patients without depression display that the two median lines have a far distance between two groups [see Fig. 1(a)]. Therefore, PSDS has a good discriminate validity that could be used to distinguish the depression patients after stroke.

The Spearman's rank correlation coefficients between every item and total score of PSDS is listed in Table 3. All the items correlated with the total score significantly ($r < 0.49$; $P < 0.001$). The value shows that PSDS has good internal consistency. The Spearman rank correlation coefficients of decreased Speech, easy fatigability, feeling of decreased capability and feeling of difficult to recover were larger than 0.6 with the total score, so these four items were thought to be the specific characteristics of poststroke depression patients. Easy to cry, insomnia, waking up too early, suicidal ideation and more irritable than usual were the general characteristics of post-stroke depression patients. Furthermore, we calculated the relevant between the score of characteristic items and HDRS to verify our hypothesis. The Spearman rank coefficient indicated a significant relevant of 0. 718 (P<0. 001). From Fig. 1(b), we can see that the correlation is relevant directly and has higher correlation in the range of minor to serve.

Table 3　The result of spearman rank correlation of PSDS

	Decreased speech	Easy fatigability	Easy to cry	Insomnia, waking up too early	Feeling of decreased capability	Suicidal ideation	Feeling of difficult to recover	More irritable than usual	PSDS (score)
Decreased-speech	1. 000	0. 356	0. 272	0. 119	0. 401	0. 209	0. 293	0. 316	0. 644
Easy fatigability	—	1. 000	0. 193	0. 285	0. 337	0. 125	0. 314	0. 174	0. 603
Easy to cry	—	—	1. 000	0. 125	0. 288	0. 450	0. 268	0. 210	0. 511
Insomnia, waking up too early	—	—	—	1. 000	0. 265	0. 135	0. 084	0. 210	0. 503
Feeling of decreased capability	—	—	—	—	1. 000	0. 212	0. 394	0. 171	0. 700
Suicidal ideation	—	—	—	—	—	1. 000	0. 382	0. 250	0. 490
Feeling of difficult to recover	—	—	—	—	—	—	1. 000	0. 302	0. 640
More irritable than usual	—	—	—	—	—	—	—	1. 000	0. 504

3. 4　Cut-off value

The cut-off value of PSDS was 6 by the ROC curves. While, the cut-off values of minor, middle and severe degree were 6, 15, and 17. Fig. 1(c) demonstrates the ROC curves of PSDS and HDRS. Short dotted line is the curves of PSDS and long dotted line is the curves of HDRS. From Fig. 1(c), we can see

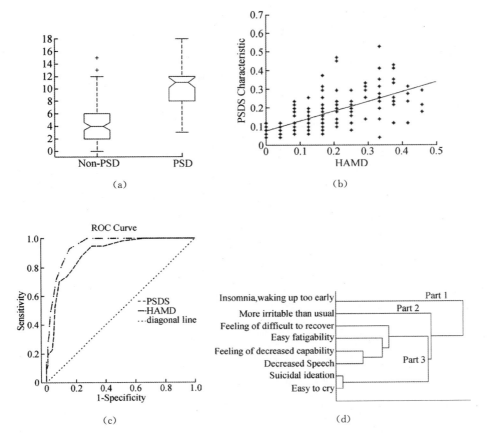

Fig. 1 (a) The box plots of patients with and without depression after stroke, the result of Kruskal – Wallis test showed a significant difference between two group (PSD and non-PSD, $P<0.001$). (b) The Spearman rank coefficient between specific characteristics of post-stroke depression patients (the score of decreased speech, easy fatigability, feeling of decreased capability and feeling of difficult to recover) and HDRS indicated a significant relevant of 0.718 ($P<0.001$). (c) ROC curve for PSDS and HDRS which areas under the line were 0.894 ($P<0.001$; 95% CI, 0.845 – 0.943) and 0.944 ($P<0.001$; 95% CI, 0.911 – 0.977). (d) The PSDS was divided into three parts by clustering analysis. PSD: post-stroke depression, non-PSD: stroke patients without depression, PSDS: Post-Stroke Depression Scale, HDRS: Hamilton Depression Rating Scale, ROC: Receiver Operating Characteristic.

that HDRS has a larger area than the PSDS, but the line of PSDS is in close proximity to the line of HDRS. The PSDS and HDRS areas under the line were 0. 894 ($P<$0. 001; 95% CI, 0. 845~0. 943) and 0. 944 ($P<$ 0. 001; 95% CI, 0. 911~0. 977). The result shows that PSDS has a good diagnostic accurate.

In the process of setting the cut-off value of PSDS, we used the one-to-one correspondence and the average method. As shown in Table 4, HDRS's cut-off value 7. 5 corresponded to the maximum Youden Index 0. 772; 6. 5 corresponded to the second Youden Index 0. 747; 7 was the average of 7. 5 and 6. 5. We calculated the cut-off value of PSDS in the light of the same method. On the other hand, the values of 15 and 17 indicate the level of middle and severe PSD according to ROC curve. Based on the cut-off values of PSDS, there were 49 patients with minor depression, 4 patients with middle depression and 1 patient with severe depression. Similarly, based on the cut-off value of HDRS, the number of patients was 51, 5 and 1 with minor to severe (see Table 5).

Table 4　Cut-off value of PSDS and HDRS

Cut-off value	PSDS			HDRS		
	Sensitivity	Specificity	Youden Index	Sensitivity	Specificity	Youden Index
1. 50	1. 000	0. 198	0. 198	—	—	—
2. 50	1. 000	0. 337	0. 337	1. 000	0. 208	0. 208
3. 50	0. 982	0. 485	0. 467	1. 000	0. 317	0. 317
4. 50	0. 947	0. 614	0. 561	1. 000	0. 525	0. 525
5. 50	0. 947	0. 693	0. 640	1. 000	0. 723	0. 723
6. 50	0. 877	0. 762	0. 639	0. 965	0. 782	0. 747
7. 50	0. 789	0. 822	0. 611	0. 930	0. 842	0. 772
8. 50	0. 737	0. 861	0. 598	0. 825	0. 891	0. 716
9. 50	0. 702	0. 911	0. 613	0. 719	0. 931	0. 650

Cut-off value	PSDS			HDRS		
	Sensitivity	Specificity	Youden Index	Sensitivity	Specificity	Youden Index
10.50	0.526	0.941	0.467	0.596	0.950	0.546
11.50	0.316	0.950	0.266	0.491	0.970	0.461
12.50	0.228	0.960	0.188	0.368	0.980	0.348
13.50	0.193	0.990	0.183	0.333	0.980	0.313
14.50	0.123	0.990	0.113	0.263	0.990	0.253
15.50	0.088	1	0.088	0.175	0.990	0.165
16.50	0.053	1	0.053	0.158	1	0.158
17.50	0.018	1	0.018			
18.50	—	—	—	0.123	1	0.123
20.00	—	—	—	0.105	1	0.105
21.50	—	—	—	0.070	1	0.070
22.50	—	—	—	0.053	1	0.053
23.50	—	—	—	0.035	1	0.035
25.50	—	—	—	0.018	1	0.018
28.00	—	—	—	0.000	1	0

Table 5   The accordance rate of PSDS and HDRS

	PSDS	HDRS
Group ($n\%$)		
Depression	54(94.74)	57(100)
Non-depression	3(5.26)	0(0)
Type of depression ($n\%$)		
None	3(5.26)	0(0)
Minor	49(85.97)	51(89.47)
Middle	4(8.77)	5(8.77)
Severe	1(1.75)	1(1.75)

To verify the effective of cut-off value, we fitted the HDRS and the PSDS by the multiple linear regression method. We can see that the 57 depressive patients' scores were all above 7, but 3 patients is less than 6 score, and PSDS accordance rate is 94.7% (Table 5). Furthermore, the PSDS cut-off value is used to 101 patients without depression, the accordance rate is 89%. PSDS plays a good auxiliary diagnostic role and distinguishes the symptom of depression excellently.

3.5 The main factors of PSDS

Fig. 1(d) shows the result of clustering analysis extracting the factors of post-stroke depression. 8 items were divided into three parts. Part 1 was insomnia, waking up too early; Part 2 was more irritable than usual; Part 3 included 6 factors that is feeling of difficult to recover, easy fatigability, feeling of decreased capability, decreased speech, easy to cry and suicidal ideation. Therefore, Part 1 was named as sleeping factors; Part 2 was named as mood factors; Part 3 was named as regressive factors.

4 Discussion

The aim of our study presents two folds: (1) draft a new specific self-rating scale screening for post-stroke depression patients; (2) verified the reliability and validity and obtained the cut-off value of the new PSDS scale.

The power of test ($1-\beta$) calculated by PASS demonstrated between 88% and 98% while sample is 158 which showed a significant difference as well as an effective result.

Although DSM-IV criteria for mood disorders have been often used to diagnose post-stroke depression (Robinson, 2003), this approach may have been misleading because some symptoms considered as diagnostic of depression can frequently occur also in patients without depression. Psychomotor retardation, fatigue, sleep, and appetite disturbance, may be a consequence of the stroke event and not necessarily indicative of depression. In particularly, previous study showed that reports of somatic complaints were not useful indicators of depression in elderly stroke patients (Gordon and Hibbard, 1991). However, fewer study attempts to revise the diagnosed criteria. In the present study, it was modified based on DSM- IV that at least two depressive symptoms excepting one core criterion symptoms of depressed mood either loss of interest or pleasure and duration of at least 1 week compared with five symptoms besides one core criterion during the same 2-week period.

Furthermore, the cognitive impairment of post-stroke depression patients may limit a patient's ability to describe or pour their anguish (Tilanus and Timmerman, 2005). In the previous study we found that memory, orientation, language and attention are the most likely impaired cognitive domains after a stroke (Tatemichi et al. , 1994). So the evaluation of the cognitive efficacy of the participants is important, and it also guarantees greater strength of the relation between questionnaire answers and the effective psychological outcome of the patient. In order to avoid the influence of cognitive impairment, the patients enrolled in our study had no complain of cognitive impairment, in addition we also interviewed with the family dependents of patients aimed to know the state of their emotional expression. Then we evaluate the cognitive function by Montreal Cognitive assessment (MoCA) and the result showed that MoCA had less influence on PSDS than HDRS (see Supplementary material).

Results of the present study are relative comprehensive from several aspects. It is also specific scale similar to post-stroke depression rating scale which is an observer-rating scale in previous preliminary report, as to the nature of the major form of poststroke depression (Gainotti et al. , 1995). First, the reliability and validity showed a good inter-consistency which is security of the diagnosis, Cronbach α and spearman rank correlation could illustrate the effective of PSDS. Second, the cut-off value was estimated. The area of PSDS was enough to show its rational index of the whole diagnostic precision of the test. We also calculated the number of minor, middle and severe level of PSDS and compared the rate with HDRS. The HDRS appears similar to self-rating scales in terms of the accurate screening for the presence of depression after stroke. Three terms of insomnia focused on the somatic aspects significantly inflated scores of HSRS. Moreover, in terms of post-stroke depression individuals, a cut-off score of 10 of this scale has been recommended as indicative of presence of depression rather than the usual 7 because of high proportion of some items (Agrell and Dehlin, 1989). However, its usefulness as a screening tool is limited by long time consuming, more factors construct and the level of examiner expertise required. Results obtained by HDRS are linked closely to the expertise of the interviewer (McDowell and Newell, 1996). In hence, the self-rating scale PSDS may be widely used to screen of the stroke patients especially the motor aphasia patients. It may benefit the patient's functional recovery, improvement the life quality and reintegration into the society ultimately by screening the depression and timely treatment.

In addition, the items of scale were clustered and fitted to find the characteristics of post-stroke depression patients. The PSDS was divided into three parts, which were named as sleeping factor, mood factors and regressive factors. Regressive characteristics contain 6 factors reflecting the decreased ability of competent and social adapt function. Differential anatomical substrates of two different subtypes of post-stroke depression: "apathetic" and "affective" one (Hama et al. , 2007). This approach has been widely criticized mainly because of the controversies in assimilating poststroke depression to endogenous mood disorders (Gordon and Hibbard, 1991). Decreased speech, easy fatigability, feeling of decreased capability and feeling of difficult to recover were listed to the suspected characteristics of post-stroke depression according to the result of Spearman rank coefficient and clustering analysis. In our opinion, even if our results uncertainty at all, however, it could lead to an updated model for the pathogenesis of post-stroke depression.

The present work was an exploratory study, technical and biological limitations inevitably exist. First, this was a crosssectional study with a relatively small sample size, the larger sample were needed to verity the results. Second, the PSDS should be used in different fields according to sex, age and side-lesion. Thirdly, the cut off value calculated by ROC curve maybe react the severity of the disease to some extent, but it is not absolute.

Overall, post-stroke depression is a common sequel of stroke that is associated with reduced functional recovery, social outcomes, quality of life and increased mortality. Early screening and assessment can lead to a significant, positive impact on the individual recovery. Reconsidering the diagnosis and finding a reliable and validity scale specifically devised to assess post-stroke depression patients is the main purpose of this study. We are optimistic about the utility of this new scale. However, as required in the development of any scale, an ongoing work to evaluate this scale and to explore the generalizability of the results in one population to other stroke populations is needed. We hope that this scale may be helpful for screening depression patients after stroke then promote early discovery and timely treatment.

5 Contributors

The order of authorship is Yingying Yue, Rui Liu, Jian Lu, Xiaojing Wang, Shining Zhang, Aiqin Wu, Qiao Wang, Yonggui Yuan. We thank to all individuals who participate in this study.

5.1 Role of funding source

The funding source had no further role in study design, in the collection, analysis and interpretation of data, in the writing of the report, and in the decision to submit the paper for publication.

5.2 Conflict of interest

No conflict declared.

5.3 Acknowledgments

We wish to thank all the participants in this study. This research was funded by Jiangsu Provincial Special Program of Medical Science (BL2012025, Yonggui Yuan).

6 Appendix A. Supplementary material

Supplementary data associated with this article can be found in the online version at http://dx.doi.org/10.1016/j.jad.2014.11.031.

References

[1] Aben, I., Verhey, F., Honig, A., Looder, J., Lousberg, R., Maes, M., 2001. Research into the specificity of depression after stroke: a review on an unresolved issue. Prog. Neuro-Psychopharmacol. Biol. Psychiatry 18, 671 – 689.

[2] Aben, I., Verhey, F., Lousberg, R., Lodder, J., Honing, A., 2002. Validity of the Beck Depression Inventory, Hospital Anxiety and Depression Scale, SCL-90,

Hamilton Depression Rating Scales screening instruments for depression in stroke patients. Psychosomatics 43, 386 – 393.

[3] Agrell, B. , Dehlin, O. , 1989. Comparison of six depression rating scales in geriatric stroke patients. Stroke 20, 1190 – 1194.

[4] American Psychiatric Association, 1994. Diagnostic and Statistical Manual of Mental Disorders—DSM-IV. American Psychiatric Press, Washington, DC. Arruda, J. E. , Stern, R. A. , Somerville, J. A. , 1999. Measurement of mood status in stroke patients: validation of the visual analogue mood scales. Arch. Phys. Med. Rehabil. 80, 676 – 680.

[5] Beck, A. T. , Ward, C. H. , Mendelson, M. , Mock, J. , Erbaugh, J. , 1961. An inventory for measuring depression. Arch. Gen. Psychiatry 4, 561 – 571.

[6] Benaim, C. , Cailly, B. , Perennou, D. , Pelissier, J. , 2004. Validation of the Aphasic Depression Rating Scale. Stroke 35, 1692 – 1696.

[7] Bjerg, B. B. , Bjerg, B. E. , Lauritzen, L. , Vilmar, T. , Bech, P. , 1997. Poststroke patients in rehabilitation: the relationship between biological impairment (CT scanning), physical disability and clinical depression. Eur. Psychiatry 12, 399 – 404.

[8] Colasanti, V. , Marianetti, M. , Micacchi, F. , Amabile, G. A. , Mina, C. , 2010. Tests for the evaluation of depression in the elderly: a systematic review. Arch. Gerontol. Geriatr. 50, 227 – 230.

[9] de Man-van Ginkel, J. M. , Hafsteinsdottir, T. , Lindeman, E. , Burger, H. , Grobbee, D. , Schuurmans, M. , 2012. An efficient way to detect poststroke depression by subsequent administration of a 9-item and a 2-item Patient Health Questionnaire. Stroke 43, 854 – 856.

[10] de Man-van Ginkel, J. M. , Hafsteinsdottir, T. B. , Lindeman, E. , Ettema, R. G. , Grobbee, D. E. , Schuurmans, M. J. , 2013. In-hospital risk prediction for post-stroke depression development and validation of the Post-stroke Depression Prediction Scale. Stroke 44, 2441 – 2445.

[11] Duncan, P. W. , Wallace, D. , Lai, S. M. , Johnson, D. , Embretson, S. , Laster, L. J. , 1999. The stroke impact scale version 2. 0. Evaluation of reliability, validity, and sensitivity to change. Stroke 30, 2131 – 2140.

[12] Fluss, R. , Faraggi, D. , Reiser, B. , 2005. Estimation of the Youden Index and its associated cutoff point. Biom. J. 47, 458 – 472.

[13] Gabaldon, L. , Fuentes, B. , Frank-Garcia, A. , Diez-Tejedor, E. , 2007. Post stroke depression: importance of its detection and treatment. Cerebrovasc. Dis. 24, 181 – 188.

[14] Gainotti, G. , Azzoni, A. , Lanzillotta, M. , Marra, C. , Razzano, C. , 1995. Some preliminary findings concerning a new scale for the assessment of depression and related symptoms in stroke patients. Ital. J. Neurol. Sci. 16, 439 – 451.

[15] Gainotti, G. , Azzoni, A. , Razzano, C. , Lanzillotta, M. , Marra, C. , Gasparini, F. , 1997. The Post-Stroke Depression Rating Scale: a test specifically devised to investigate affective disorders of stroke patients. J. Clin. Exp. Neuropsychol. 19, 340 – 356.

[16] Gordon, W. A. , Hibbard, M. R. , 1991. Issues in the diagnosis of post-stroke depression. Rehabil. Psychol. 36, 71 – 85.

[17] Hackett, M. L. , Anderson, C. S. , 2005. Predictors of depression after stroke: a systematic review of observational studies. Stroke 36, 2296 – 2301.

[18] Hama, S. , Yamashita, H. , Shigenobu, M. , Watanabe, A. , Kurisu, K. , Yamawaki, S. , Kitaoka, T. , 2007. Post-stroke affective or apathetic depression and lesion location: left frontal lobe and bilateral basal ganglia. Eur. Arch. Psychiatry Clin. Neurosci. 257, 149 – 152.

[19] Hamilton, M. , 1960. A rating scale for depression. J. Neurol. Neurosurg. Psychiatry 23, 56 – 62.

[20] Kang, H. J. , Stewart, R. , Kim, J. M. , Jang, J. E. , Kim, S. Y. , Bae, K. Y. , Kim, S. W. , Shin, I. S. , Park, M. S. , Cho, K. H. , Yoon, J. S. , 2013. Comparative validity of depression assessment scales for screening post-stroke depression. J. Affect. Disord. 147, 186 – 191.

[21] Lincoln, N. B. , Sutcliffe, L. M. , Unsworth, G. , 2000. Validation of the Stroke Aphasic Depression Questionnaire (SADQ) for use with patients in hospital. Clin. Neuropsychol. Assess. 1, 88 – 96.

[22] Loubinoux, I. , Kronenberg, G. , Endres, M. , Schumann-Bard, P. , Freret, T. ,

Filipkowski, R. K. , Kaczmarek, L. , Popa-Wagner, A. , 2012. Post-stroke depression: mechanisms, translation and therapy. J. Cell. Mol. Med. 16, 1961 – 1969.

[23] Mahoney, F. I. , Barthel, D. W. , 1965. Functional evaluation: the Barthel Index. Md. State Med. J. 14, 61 – 65.

[24] McCrate, R. R. , Kurtz, J. E. , Yamagata, S. , Terracciano, A. , 2011. Iternal consistency, retest reliability, and their implications for personality scale validity. Personal. Soc. Psychol. Rev. 15, 28 – 50.

[25] McDowell, I. , Newell, C. , 1996. Measuring Health. A Guide to Rating Scales and Questionnaires, NewYork, 2nd ed. Oxford University Press. Montgomery, S. A. , Asberg, M. , 1979. A new depression scale designed to be sensitive to change. Br. J. Psychiatry 134, 382 – 389.

[26] Park, H. M. , 2008. Hypothesis Testing and Statistical Power of a Test. Working Paper. The University Information Technology Services (UITS) Center for Statistical and Mathematical Computing, Indiana University.

[27] Pompili, M. , Venturini, P. , Campi, S. , Seretti, M. E. , Montebovi, F. , Lamis, D. A. , Serafini, G. , Amore, M. , Girardi, P. , 2012. Do stroke patients have an increased risk of developing suicidal ideation or dying by suicide? An overview of the current literature. CNS Neurosci. Ther. 18, 711 – 721.

[28] Rosner, B. , 2004. Fundamentals of Biostatistics, Seventh Edition Harvard University, Canada.

[29] Radloff, L. S. , 1977. The CES-D scale: a self-report depression scale for research in the general population. Appl. Psychol. Meas. 1, 385 – 401.

[30] Robinson, R. G. , 2003. Poststroke depression: prevalence, diagnosis, treatment, and disease progression. Biol. Psychiatry 54, 376 – 387.

[31] Salter, K. , Bhogal, S. K. , Foley, N. , Jutai, J. , Teasell, R. , 2007. The assessment of poststroke depression. Top. Stroke Rehabil. 14, 1 – 24.

[32] Spalletta, G. , Robinson, R. G. , 2010. How should depression be diagnosed in patients with stroke? Acta Psychiatr. Scand. 121, 401 – 403.

[33] Tatemichi, T. K. , Desmond, D. W. , Stern, Y. , Paik, M. , Sano, M. , Bagiella,

E. , 1994. Cognitive impairment after stroke: frequency, patterns, and relationship to functional abilities. J. Neurol. Neurosurg. Psychiatry 57, 202 – 207.

[34] Tilanus, J. , Timmerman, L. , 2005. Poststroke depression. Rev. Clin. Gerontol. 14, 37 – 43.

[35] van Swieten, J. C. , Koudstaal, P. J. , Visser, M. C. , Schouten, H. J. , van Gijn, J. , 1988. Inter observer agreement for the assessment of handicap in stroke patients. Stroke 19, 604 – 607.

[36] Williams, L. S. , Brizendine, E. J. , Plue, L. , Bakas, T. , Tu, W. , Hendrie, H. , Kroenke, K. , 2005. Performance of the PHQ-9 as a screening tool for depression after stroke. Stroke 36, 635 – 638.

[37] Yesavage, J. A. , Brink, T. L. , Rose, T. L. , Lum, O. , Huang, V. , Adey, M. , Leirer, V. O. , 1983. Development and validation of a geriatric depression screening scale: a preliminary report. J. Psychiatr. Res. 17, 37 – 49.

[38] Zhang, N. , Wang, C. X. , Wang, A. X. , Bai, Y. , Zhou, Y. , Wang, Y. L. , Zhang, T. , Zhou, J. , Yu, X. , Sun, X. Y. , Liu, Z. R. , Zhao, X. Q. , Wang, Y. J. , Prospective Cohort study on Incidence and Outcome of Patients with Poststroke Depression in China (PRIOD) Investigators, 2012. Time course of depression and one-year prognosis of patients with stroke in mainland China. CNS Neurosci. Ther. 18, 475 – 481.

[39] Zigmond, A. S. , Snaith, R. P. , 1983. The Hospital Anxiety and Depression Scale. Acta Psychiatr. Scand. 67, 361 – 370.

[40] Zung, A. , 1965. A self-rating depression scale. Arch. Gen. Psychiatry 12, 63 – 70.

[作者及发表刊物:

Yingying Yue, Rui Liu, Jian Lu, Xiaojing Wang, Shining Zhang, Aiqin Wu, Qiao Wang, Yonggui Yuan. Reliability and Validity of a new post-stroke depression scale in Chinese population[J]. Journal of Affective Disorders, 2015,174:317 – 323.]

卒中后抑郁障碍评估量表(PSDS)

指导语:请仔细阅读每一条,把意思弄明白,然后根据您最近一星期的实际情况,选择最适合您的答案。

圈出最适合你情况的分数				
1. 言语减少(不想说话)	0	1	2	3
2. 容易疲乏	0	1	2	3
3. 容易哭泣	0	1	2	3
4. 睡眠差、早醒	0	1	2	3
5. 感到自己能力下降	0	1	2	3
6. 有想死的念头	0	1	2	3
7. 感觉自己好不了	0	1	2	3
8. 比平常容易生气激动	0	1	2	3

(0=无;1=小部分时间有;2=相当多时间有;3=绝大部分或全部时间有)

另:英文版卒中后抑郁障碍评估量表

Post-stroke depression scale (PSDS)

Please read each statement carefully and decide how much of the time the statement describes according to your feeling after well understand during the last seven days.

Select the most appropriate statement				
1. Decreased speech (don't want to speak)	0	1	2	3
2. Easy fatigability	0	1	2	3
3. Easy to cry	0	1	2	3
4. Insomnia, waking up too early	0	1	2	3
5. Feeling of decreased capability	0	1	2	3
6. Suicidal ideation	0	1	2	3
7. Feeling of difficult to recover	0	1	2	3
8. More irritable than usual	0	1	2	3

Note: Each question is scored on a scale of 0 through 3;0=absent, 1=some of the time, 2=part of the time, 3=most of the time.

The reliability and validity of a Chinese-version Short Health Anxiety Inventory: an investigation of university students

Background: The Short Health Anxiety Inventory (SHAI) is widely used in English-speaking populations, with good reliability and validity. For further research needs in the Chinese population, it was translated into a Chinese version (CSHAI). Furthermore, the reliability, validity, and cutoff score were examined in a nonclinical population in the People's Republic of China.

Methods: Three hundred and sixteen undergraduates were evaluated by a set of questionnaires including CSHAI, Zung Self-Rating Anxiety Scale (SAS), Zung Self-Rating Depression Scale (SDS), and the State-Trait Anxiety Inventory (STAI). Fifty-eight students completed CSHAI again after 30 days.

Results: The two-factor model had satisfactory fit indices. The correlation coefficients between each item with the CSHAI total and each subscale were between 0.386 and 0.779. The Cronbach's alpha coefficients of CSHAI total and its subscales were 0.742, 0.743, and 0.788, respectively, and the split-half coefficients were 0.757, 0.788, and 0.912. The test-retest correlation coefficients were, respectively, 0.598 ($P \leqslant 0.001$), 0.539 ($P \leqslant 0.001$), and 0.691 ($P \leqslant 0.001$). Convergent validities were respectively 0.389—0.453, 0.389—0.410, and 0.250—0.401, and discriminant validities were -5.689 ($P \leqslant 0.001$), -5.614 ($P \leqslant 0.001$), and -3.709 ($P \leqslant 0.001$). The cutoff score was 15.

Conclusion: CSHAI showed good factor structure, reliability, convergent validity, and discriminant validity, and 15 was determined to be the appropriate cutoff score for screening health anxiety.

Keywords: health anxiety, confirmatory factor analysis, cutoff score

中 文 摘 要

中文版简式健康焦虑量表的信效度研究

张钰群　刘　瑞　李国宏　毛圣芹　袁勇贵

研究背景：简式健康焦虑量表（Short Health Anxiety Inventory，SHAI）应用广泛且具有良好的评价指标，而其在中国人群中尚未被应用。本研究制定了适用于中国人群的中文版 SHAI（Chinese SHAI，CSHAI），并对 CSHAI 的信度和效度进行了验证。

方法：2 名研究生将 SHAI 翻译成中文后再次转译为英文，会议商讨 CSHAI 是否适用于中国人群，修改后由精神科专家确定最终版本。对 316 名大学生进行一系列量表的评估，包括 CSHAI、宗氏焦虑自评量表（Zung Self-rating Anxiety Scale，SAS）、宗氏抑郁自评量表（Zung Self-rating Depression Scale，SDS）和状态特质焦虑量表（State-Trait Anxiety Inventory，STAI）。时隔 30 天，58 名学生再次完成 CSHAI 的评估。

结果：每个条目与 CSHAI 及分量表的相关系数在 0.386 和 0.779 之间。CSHAI 总分及分量表的 α 系数分别为 0.742，0.743 和 0.788，分半系数分别为 0757，0.788 和 0.912。CSHAI 总分及分量表的重测系数分别为 0.598（$P<0.001$），0.539（$P<0.001$）和 0.691（$P<0.001$）。CSHAI 总分及分量表的聚合效度分别为 0.389～0.453，0.389～0.410 和 0.250～0.401，判别效度分别为 -5.689（$P<0.001$），-5.614（$P<0.001$）和 -3.709（$P<0.001$）。上述结果证明 CSHAI 双因素模型拟合指数较高。CSHAI 总分的阈值分数为 15 分。

结论：CSHSI 具备良好的因子结构及信效度；受试者 CSHAI 总分 15 分及以上可考虑为健康焦虑。

关键词：中文版简式健康焦虑量表；验证性因子分析；信效度；阈值

1 Introduction

Health anxiety (HA) refers to a negative interpretation and fears a-bout the meaning of both ordinary and unusual bodily sensations.[1] The prevalence in the general population varies,[2-4] and it considerably reduces life quality and increases the chance of medical consultation and seeking of psychotherapeutic or psychiatric treatment.[5,6] Hypochondriasis is consid-ered an extreme form of HA;[7] however, HA and hypochondriasis are not distinguished clearly.[2-4] Actually, hypochondriasis and HA share a com-mon component of phobia (and, more broadly, health-and disease-related concerns), but that does not seem to be the case with disease conviction, as definitions of HA usually do not include an idea or belief that a serious ill-ness is present.[8] This results in various measurements for HA, including the Illness Attitudes Scale (IAS), Whiteley Index (WI), Structured Diag-nostic Interview for Hypochondriasis (SDIH),[9] and Short Health Anxiety Inventory (SHAI).[10]

Salkovskis et al[10] developed the Health Anxiety Inventory (HAI) (64 items) and a shortened version of this scale, the SHAI (18 items). The shortened version was sensitive to both normal levels of health concern and severe HA. In addition, SHAI was demonstrated to be an appropriate measurement that was sensitive to both mild and more severe forms of HA in both medical and nonmedical samples.[11] Adequate-to-excellent internal consistency in undergraduate students and strong construct validity was af-firmed.[12] The factor structure,[13-15] reliability and validity, cutoff score, versions in different languages, and various populations have been exam-ined. The original factorial structure of SHAI included a two-factor mod-el[10,11,15] and a three-factor model.[16] The results of the above investigations are inconsistent, varying with the number of items. Nevertheless, the two-factor structure of SHAI has received the greatest support and can provide a more comprehensive assessment of the factor structure of HA.

The English-version SHAI has been widely explored, mainly in English-speaking populations. Just one study, with a sample of 832 Spanish secondary school adolescents, used the Spanish version. [17] The results indicated adequate reliability of the inventory and suggested SHAI may be considered an appropriate instrument for assessing HA in Spanish-speaking adolescents. In Asian countries, there is as yet no appropriate measurement for screening HA either in clinical samples or nonclinical populations. The Zung Self-Rating Anxiety Scale (SAS) is the most widely used measure in the People's Republic of China for screening anxiety. [18-20] The main aim of this study was to analyze the reliability and validity of SHAI for its possible use in assessing HA in Chinese general populations. The second aim was to explore the cutoff score of the Chinese-version SHAI (CSHAI).

2 Methods

2.1 Participants

Three hundred and sixteen healthy medical students (aged from 18 to 27 years) participated in this study. There were 122 men (mean age 21.69 years with standard deviation [SD] 1.56, range 19 to 26) and 194 women (mean age 21.76 years with SD 1.72, range 18 to 27). There was no significant age difference between the two sex groups ($t=-0.387$; 95% confidence interval [CI]: $-0.45 \sim 0.30$; $P=0.699$). Another 61 students participated in the test − retest reliability research and they completed the CSHAI twice every 30 days. Finally, 17 men (mean age 22.88 years with SD 1.27, range 20 to 25) and 41 women (mean age 21.88 years with SD

1. 52, range 20 to 27) were retained. There was a significant age difference between the two sex groups ($t=2.397$; 95% CI: 0.16~1.84; $P=0.02$) either. All participants were confirmed to have no history of serious illness (including mental disorders and neurological diseases).

2.2 Measures

The participants were asked to fill in the following four Chinese-version questionnaires.

2.3 CSHAI

The CSHAI[10] has two factors, corresponding to: 1) the feared likelihood of becoming ill (Illness Likelihood [IL], 14 items), and 2) the feared negative consequences of becoming ill (Negative Consequences [NC], four items). Each item of the CSHAI consists of four statements that range from "I do not" (0) to "I spend most of my time" (3). The total scores are from 0 to 54.

2.4 The Zung Self-Rating Anxiety Scale

Zung compiled the Self-Rating Anxiety Scale (SAS) in 1971, and it is a 20-item, self-report measure of anxious symptoms.[21] Each of the items is ranked on a four-point Likert scale, ranging from "never occurring" or "a little of the time" to "most of the time". Responses were summed to calculate a total score, with higher scores indicating greater levels of anxious symptomatology. Good validity has been demonstrated for the Chinese version of SAS.[22] Standard scores above 50 suggest clinically significant levels of anxiety in a Chinese population.[22]

2.5 The Zung Self-Rating Depression Scale

The Zung Self-Rating Depression Scale (SDS)[23] is a 20-item self-report tool which was developed to measure depressive symptoms and for depression screening. In a study of the Chinese-version SDS in students,[24] good internal consistency was confirmed, with a Pearson's correlation coefficient of 0.313~0.640.

2.6 The State-Trait Anxiety Inventory

The State-Trait Anxiety Inventory (STAI)[25] is a 40-item measure of anxiety. It can measure both state anxiety (how anxious a person is feeling at a particular moment [S-AI]) and trait anxiety (how dispositionally anxious a person is across time and situations [T-AI]) and consists of two separate subscales containing 20 items each. Each item is scored from 1 to 4, with the total score ranging from 20 to 80 for each scale and high scores indicating increased anxiety. Good test-retest reliability has been demonstrated,[25] with a Pearson's correlation coefficient of 0.73~0.77 in S-AI and 0.31~0.33 in T-AI.

2.7 Procedures

The SHAI was translated by two master's students, and a physician proficient in English without access to the original English version performed back-translation. Then, a meeting was held to discuss each item's suitability for a Chinese population. Finally, two psychiatrists checked the translated version and agreed upon the primary version of CSHAI. A pilot test of the Chinese-language survey was conducted with 30 participants. There were no reports of misunderstandings, so this version was used as the final version.

The participants in this study were adult volunteer university students. Three hundred and sixteen students filled out the paper-based questionnaires anonymously over 2 days, and the entire procedure took approximately 20~30 minutes. Fifty-eight students completed the CSHAI twice, with an interval of 30 days before the second instance. The students did not receive an academic or other reward for participation. The study procedure was approved by the ethical committee of Zhongda Hospital, which is affiliated to Southeast University (Nanjing, People's Republic of China).

2.8 Analyses

To complete the analyses, the Predictive Analytics Software (PASW) Statistics 18 package and IBM SPSS Amos 22 were used (IBM Corporation, Armonk, NY, USA). The factor structure of the CSHAI was confirmed following the Bentler and Bonett[26] criteria, using three commonly used indices: comparative fit index (CFI), root mean-square error of approximation (RMSEA), and Satorra-Bentler chi-square. The value of CFI should exceed a recommended cutoff value of 0.90 (more liberal) or 0.95 (more strict), and a value of RMSEA less than 0.08 (more liberal) or 0.05 (more strict) indicates a good fit. [27] Internal consistency was assessed with the Cronbach's alpha coefficient and split-half coefficient. Convergent validity was documented using a Pearson's correlation coefficient by comparing the CSHAI total with the SAS. Comparison between the anxiety group and nonanxiety group was analyzed by independent-samples t-test. P-values less than 0.05 were considered to indicate statistical significance.

The cutoff score was determined by the Youden index, combining the sensitivity value and specificity value[28] that resulted from the receiver operating characteristic (ROC) curve. The areas of ROC curve could be used as an index to examine the precision of the test. The Youden index was calculated by the following formula:

$$\text{Youden index} = \text{sensitivity value} + \text{specificity value} - 1 \qquad (1)$$

The maximum of the Youden index is the best cutoff value. To verify the accuracy and effectiveness of this cutoff value, we calculated the accordance rate compared with SAS and used multiple linear regression to observe the comparison directly.

3 Results

3.1 Confirmatory factor analysis

Standardized loadings are shown in Table 1 and the confirmatory factor analysis model in Figure S1. All item loadings were high, with one exception: item 10 for IL. Indices for the original two factors, $\chi^2 (134) = 274.282$, $P \leqslant 0.001$, CFI$=0.901$, and RMSEA$=0.058$, indicated a good fit.

Table 1　Confirmatory factor analysis: factor loadings (N=316)

SHAI item	IL[a] (items 1~14)	NC[a] (items 15~18)
1	0.581	
2	0.345	
3	0.348	
4	0.616	
5	0.762	
6	0.655	
7	0.590	
8	0.475	
9	0.556	
10	0.277	
11	0.663	
12	0.677	
13	0.368	
14	0.355	
15		0.608
16		0.586
17		0.701
18		0.556

Note: [a]A subscale of CSHAI.

Abbreviations: CSHAI, Chinese-Version Short Health Anxiety Inventory; Il, Illness Likelihood; NC, Negative Consequences.

3.2 Internal consistency

Table S1 shows correlations of the CSHAI total with IL, NC, and each item, as determined by Pearson's correlation coefficient. The coefficient of determination ranged from 0.392 to 0.700 for each item ($P \leqslant 0.01$), 0.965 for IL ($P \leqslant 0.01$), and 0.731 for NC ($P \leqslant 0.01$). In addition, the correlation coefficient of IL with items 1 to 14 ranged from 0.417 to 0.730 ($P \leqslant 0.01$). Moreover, NC with items 15 to 18 ranged from 0.651 to 0.780 ($P \leqslant 0.01$). The remarkably high coefficient between CSHAI and each item indicated the high consistency of CSHAI. The correlation between both factors was identified as moderate (0.526), indicating that they are related but measure different aspects of HA.

The analysis of the internal consistency of the CSHAI total generated a Cronbach's alpha coefficient of 0.742. The coefficients for the IL and NC subscales were 0.743 and 0.788. The split-half coefficients of the CSHAI total, IL, and NC were 0.757, 0.788, and 0.912, respectively.

3.3 Test – retest reliability

For the 58 participants who completed the CSHAI twice, Pearson's correlation coefficient was 0.560 for CSHAI total ($P \leqslant 0.01$), 0.438 for IL ($P \leqslant 0.01$), and 0.720 ($P \leqslant 0.01$) for NC, indicating a relatively satisfactory level of test – retest reliability.

3.4 Convergent validity

The correlations of CSHAI with SAS, SDS, S-AI, and T-AI are presented in Table 2. CSHAI total was significantly correlated with SAS ($r = 0.390$, $P \leqslant 0.01$), S-AI ($r = 0.429$, $P \leqslant 0.01$), and T-AI ($r = 0.454$, $P \leqslant 0.01$). On the contrary, the correlation of CSHAI with SDS was not significant ($r = 0.078$, $P > 0.05$). Similar to CSHAI total, IL and NC were also significantly correlated with SAS, S-AI, and T-AI.

Table 2　Correlations of SHAI with other scales

	SAS	SDS	S-AI	T-AI
SHAI total	0.389**	0.077	0.428**	0.453**
IL[a]	0.389**	0.086	0.391**	0.410**
NC[a]	0.250**	0.027	0.369**	0.401**

Notes: Data presented as Pearson's correlation coefficient (r). [a]A subscale of SHAI, SAI and T-AI are subscales of STAI. ** $P \leqslant 0.001$.

Abbreviations: SHAI, Short Health Anxiety Inventory; Il, Illness Likelihood; NC, Negative Consequences; SAS, Zung Self-Rating Anxiety Scale; SDS, Self-Rating Depression Scale; SAI, State Anxiety; T-AI, trait anxiety; STai, state-Trait anxiety inventory.

3.5　Discriminant validity

Three hundred and sixteen participants were divided into two groups according to the cutoff score of 50 SAS standard scores. There were 39 students in the anxiety group (accounting for 12.34%) and 277 in the non-anxiety group (accounting for 87.66%) (see Table 3). Comparing CSHAI scores, we found that there were significant differences between the anxiety and non-anxiety group.

Table 3　comparison of CSHAI scores between students in the anxiety group and non-anxiety group

	Non-anxiety group($N=277$)	Anxiety group($N=39$)	t
SHAI total	11.28±5.43	16.97±8.27	−5.689**
IL[a]	9.03±4.37	13.54±6.62	−5.614**
NC[a]	2.26±1.77	3.44±2.35	−3.709**

Notes: [a]Data presented as mean±standard deviation. a subscale of CSHAI. ** $P \leqslant 0.001$.
Abbreviations: CSHAI, chinese-version Short Health Anxiety Inventory; IL, Illness Likelihood; NC, Negative Consequences.

3.6　Cutoff value of CSHAI

The cutoff value of CSHAI was determined to be 15 by the ROC curve. Figure 1 demonstrates the ROC curve of CSHAI and SAS with the data of 316 students. The short dotted line is the curve of SAS and the long dotted line is the curve of CSHAI. SAS had a larger area under the curve than CSHAI, but the values were close. The area under the curve of CSHAI was 0. 745 ($P \leqslant 0.001$; 95% CI: 0. 657—0. 834) and that under SAS was 0. 993 ($P \leqslant 0.001$; 95% CI: 0—1). The results suggest that CSHAI had relatively good diagnostic accuracy.

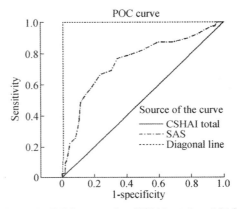

Figure 1　ROC curves for CSHAI total and SAS.

Notes: The areas under the ROC curve for SHAI and SAS were 0. 745 ($P \leqslant 0.001$; 95% CI: 0. 657—0. 834) and 0. 993 ($P \leqslant 0.001$; 95% CI: 0—1), respectively.

Abbreviations: CI, confidence interval; ROC, receiver operating characteristic; SAS, Zung Self-Rating Anxiety Scale; Cshai, Chinese-version Short Health Anxiety Inventory.

One-to-one correspondence and the average method were used while setting the cutoff value of CSHAI. Table 4 shows the SAS cutoff value of 49 corresponded to the maximum Youden index of 0. 993. The maximum Youden index of CSHAI was 0. 428 confirmed the cutoff value of CSHAI. Because of integral scores, the students with 15 or more in CSHAI total were considered to have HA. In this way, 92 students were verified to have HA, which accounted for 29. 11%. This rate was significantly different to that of the anxiety group assessed by SAS ($\chi^2 = 27.05$, $P \leqslant 0.001$).

Table 4 Cutoff Values of CSHAI and SAS

Cutoff value	CSHAI			Cutoff value	SAS		
	Sensitivity	Specificity	Youden index		Sensitivity	Specificity	Youden index
−1.00	1.000	0.000	0.000	24.00	1.000	0.000	0.000
1.00	1.000	0.014	0.014	25.50	1.000	0.018	0.018
2.50	1.000	0.036	0.036	26.50	1.000	0.032	0.032
3.50	0.974	0.054	0.029	27.50	1.000	0.054	0.054
4.50	0.974	0.072	0.047	29.00	1.000	0.105	0.105
5.50	0.949	0.119	0.068	30.50	1.000	0.177	0.177
6.50	0.923	0.162	0.086	31.50	1.000	0.235	0.235
7.50	0.897	0.224	0.121	32.50	1.000	0.300	0.300
8.50	0.872	0.318	0.189	34.00	1.000	0.361	0.361
9.50	0.872	0.408	0.280	35.50	1.000	0.433	0.433
10.50	0.821	0.502	0.322	36.50	1.000	0.509	0.509
11.50	0.795	0.570	0.365	37.50	1.000	0.570	0.570
12.50	0.769	0.657	0.426	39.00	1.000	0.661	0.661
13.50	0.692	0.693	0.385	40.50	1.000	0.715	0.715
14.50	0.667	0.762	0.428	41.50	1.000	0.776	0.776
15.50	0.590	0.812	0.402	42.50	1.000	0.819	0.819
16.50	0.538	0.852	0.390	44.00	1.000	0.874	0.874
17.50	0.487	0.884	0.372	45.50	1.000	0.921	0.921
18.50	0.359	0.895	0.254	46.50	1.000	0.957	0.957
19.50	0.256	0.917	0.173	47.50	1.000	0.978	0.978
20.50	0.231	0.942	0.173	49.00	1.000	0.993	0.993
21.50	0.231	0.949	0.180	50.50	0.872	0.993	0.865
22.50	0.128	0.968	0.096	51.50	0.795	0.993	0.788
23.50	0.103	0.975	0.077	52.50	0.615	0.993	0.608

Cutoff value	CSHAI			Cutoff value	SAS		
	Sensitivity	Specificity	Youden index		Sensitivity	Specificity	Youden index
24.50	0.103	0.978	0.081	54.00	0.462	0.993	0.454
26.00	0.026	0.982	0.008	55.50	0.410	0.993	0.403
28.00	0.026	0.989	0.015	56.50	0.333	0.993	0.326
29.50	0.026	0.993	0.018	57.50	0.256	0.993	0.249
30.50	0.026	0.996	0.022	59.00	0.179	0.993	0.172
42.50	0.026	1.000	0.026	60.50	0.128	0.993	0.121
55.00	0.000	1.000	0.000	62.00	0.077	0.996	0.073
—	—	—	—	64.00	0.051	0.996	0.048
—	—	—	—	67.50	0.000	0.996	−0.004
—	—	—	—	71.00	0.000	1.000	0.000

Abbreviations: CSHAI, Chinese-version Short Health Anxiety Inventory; SAS, Zung Self-Rating Anxiety Scale.

4 Discussion

The aim of the present study was twofold: first, to confirm the reliability and validity of the two-structure CSHAI; and, second, to analyze the cutoff score of CSHAI in students. The confirmatory factor analysis showed satisfactory fit indices, confirming that, in the students from 18 to 27 years old, the CSHAI has the same two factors as those reported by Salkovskis et al,[10] IL and NC. Moreover, it was close to the original version, with CFI=0.96 and RMSEA=0.052.

In addition, CSHAI showed relatively good reliability and validity, based on recommendations that a Cronbach's alpha coefficient over 0.80 is essential for acceptability as a basic research tool.[29] However, the alpha coefficient of the original CSHAI was 0.71 when used in a nonpatient sample, which was similar to NC, having an alpha coefficient of 0. 72. [10] This relates to the confusion of HA and hypochondriasis. HA may be a kind of symptom, but hypochondriasis is a kind of mental disorder. For nonpatients, HA screening and diagnosis is more difficult. This phenomenon is consistent with the Spanish-version CSHAI, which had low internal consistency of NC. [17] In addition, the number of items influences results. Karademas et al's investigation of students in 2008 used a 14-item SHAI, [30] and Boston and Merrick[31] investigated community adults with an 18-item SHAI. However, in patients 14-item[32] and 18-item[33, 34] model all be used. Thus, the use of NC has some controversy when screening different populations.

In this study, SAS as a measurement to screen anxiety was selected to confirm the validity of CSHAI. In a paper by Rachman, [35] HA disorder as a new kind of anxiety disorder was associated with posttraumatic stress disorder, obsessive-compulsive disorder, panic disorder, and general anxiety disorder. The validity results suggested CSHAI total and the two subscales were significantly correlated with SAS, and two student groups were significantly different in CSHAI score.

The cutoff score was calculated using the Youden index, combining the sensitivity value and specificity value that resulted from the ROC curve in a sample of 316 students. The results showed 15 was the cutoff score for diagnosing HA in students. The area under the curve was relatively accurate for diagnosing HA, though it was below perfectly accurate (area under the curve=1). [36] This finding was consistent with Tang et al's[37] study, which shows a cutoff point of 18 or higher in the SHAI reliably identifies people meeting diagnostic criteria for hypochondriasis, whilst a score between 15 and 17 represents a high level of HA but not enough to meet the diagnosis criteria of hypochondriasis. The study of Alberts et al[12] suggests a cutoff of 27 would apply, while Sulkowski et al[38] report a cutoff score as high as 38.

The controversies of cutoff value have brought some troubles to studies with CSHAI. Rachman[35] points out that severe HA, the extreme end of the continuum of HA, is often termed "hypochondriasis". Although patients with HA or hypochondriasis would have similar avoidance and safety behaviors (such as avoiding going to hospital, repeated medical consultations and tests, self-checking), beliefs differ to some extent. [39-41] Hypochondriacal beliefs are resistant to disconfirmation. Unlike HA, in which future dangers are anticipated, in hypochondriasis, the danger is present and active, and the belief is fixed. [35] The dimensional characteristics and concept confusion of these two disorders closely relate to the construct and cutoff value of CSHAI. Therefore, verifying the reliability and validity of different versions of SHAI before investigation is necessary. This study enriches the usage of CSHAI, which represents one more measure for assessing HA and, at the same time, helps physicians to discover HA faster and more conveniently.

4.1　Limitations

In this study, the participants were recruited from only one university. Previous studies select particular populations as the subjects, which would be not referenced in a general population HA study. Future study must be conducted in both general and clinical populations. Moreover, comparisons between the two-factor structure (contain IL and NC) and only IL structure of SHAI were not explored. A wider-ranging study on a larger randomized population sample should be planned for further validation in a general Chinese population. Despite these limitations, the CSHAI was demonstrated to be useful in Chinese university students and had significant correlations with scales for screening anxiety.

4. 2　Conclusion

The goal of this study was to validate CSHAI and construct a valid and reliable tool to measure HA in a Chinese population. This research confirms that CSHAI presented good internal consistency, highly satisfactory convergence, discriminant validity, and 15 as an appropriate cutoff score. It is promising for helping assessment of HA in the People's Republic of China and will enrich the pools of SHAI study.

5　Acknowledgment

We would like to thank the medical students for completion of the questionnaires.

6　Disclosure

The authors report no conflicts of interest in this work.

References

[1]　Hadjistavropoulos HD, Janzen JA, Kehler MD, Leclerc JA, Sharpe D, Bourgault-Fagnou MD. Core cognitions related to health anxiety in self-reported medical and non-medical samples. J Behav Med. 2012,35: 167 - 178.

[2]　Sunderland M, Newby JM, Andrews G. Health anxiety in Australia: prevalence, comorbidity, disability and service use. Br J Psychiatry. 2013,202:56 - 61.

[3]　Noyes R Jr, Happel RL, Yagla SJ. Correlates of hypochondriasis in a nonclinical population. Psychosomatics. 1999,40:461 - 469.

[4]　Martin A, Jacobi F. Features of hypochondriasis and illness worry in the general population in Germany. Psychosom Med. 2006,68:770 - 777.

[5]　Fink P, Ørnbøl E, Christensen KS. The outcome of health anxiety in primary care.

A two-year 24 follow-up study on health care costs and self-rated health. PLoS One. 2010,5:e9873.

[6] Creed F, Barsky A. A systematic review of the epidemiology of somatisation disorder and hypochondriasis. J Psychosom Res. 2004,56:391 – 408.

[7] Gerolimatos LA, Edelstein BA. Anxiety-related constructs mediate the relation between age and health anxiety. Aging Ment Health. 2012,16:975 – 982.

[8] Starcevic V. Hypochondriasis and health anxiety: conceptual challenges. Br J Psychiatry. 2013,202:7 – 8.

[9] Marcus DK, Gurley JR, Marchi MM, Bauer C. Cognitive and perceptual variables in hypochondriasis and health anxiety: a systematic review. Clin Psychol Rev. 2007,27:127 – 139.

[10] Salkovskis PM, Rimes KA, Warwick HM, Clark DM. The Health Anxiety Inventory: development and validation of scales for the measurement of health anxiety and hypochondriasis. Psychol Med. 2002,32: 843 – 853.

[11] Alberts NM, Sharpe D, Kehler MD, Hadjistavropoulos HD. Health anxiety: comparison of the latent structure in medical and non-medical samples. J Anxiety Disord. 2011,25:612 – 614.

[12] Alberts NM, Hadjistavropoulos HD, Jones SL, Sharpe D. The Short Health Anxiety Inventory: a systematic review and meta-analysis. J Anxiety Disord. 2013,27:68 – 78.

[13] Abramowitz JS, Olatunji BO, Deacon BJ. Health anxiety, hypochondriasis, and the anxiety disorders. Behav Ther. 2007,38:86 – 94.

[14] Olatunji BO. Incremental specificity of disgust propensity and sensitivity in the prediction of health anxiety dimensions. J Behav Ther Exp Psychiatry. 2009,40: 230 – 239.

[15] Wheaton MG, Berman NC, Franklin JC, Abramowitz JS. Health anxiety: latent structure and associations with anxiety-related psychological processes in a student sample. J Psychopathol Behav Assess. 2010,32: 565 – 574.

[16] Abramowitz JS, Deacon BJ, Valentiner DP. The Short Health Anxiety Inventory: psychometric properties and construct validity in a nonclinical sample. Cognit Ther Res. 2007,31:871 – 883.

[17] Morales A, Espada JP, Carballo JL, Piqueras JA, Orgilés M. Short health anxiety inventory: factor structure and psychometric properties in Spanish adolescents. J Health Psychol. 2015,20(2):123 – 131.

[18] Ye RF, Geng QS, Chen J, et al. Comparison of three scales to detect anxiety in general hospital outpatients: HADS, SAS and HAMA. Chinese Journal of Behavioral Medicine and Brain Science. 2013,22: 271 – 273. Chinese.

[19] Yin W, Pang L, Cao X, et al. Factors associated with depression and anxiety among patients attending community-based methadone maintenance treatment in China. Addiction. 2015,110 Suppl 1:51 – 60.

[20] Liu N, Cadilhac DA, Andrew NE, et al. Randomized controlled trial of early rehabilitation after intracerebral hemorrhage stroke: difference in outcomes within 6 months of stroke. Stroke. 2014,45:3502 – 3507.

[21] Zung WW. A rating instrument for anxiety disorders. Psychosomatics. 1971,12: 371 – 379.

[22] Wu WY. Self-Rating Anxiety Scale. In: Zhang ZJ, editor. [Behavioral Medicine Inventory Manual]. Beijing: The Chinese Medicine Electronic Audio and Video Publishing House. 2005,213 – 214. Chinese.

[23] Zung WW. A self-rating depression scale. Arch Gen Psychiatry. 1965,12:63 – 70.

[24] Zhang DX, Luo JH, Peng LZ, et al. [Factor analysis on survey results of the self-rating depression scale (SDS) in students]. Journal of Kunming Medical University. 2012,5:61 – 63. Chinese.

[25] Zhang ZJ. state-trait Anxiety Inventory. In: Zhang ZJ, editor. [Behavioral Medicine Inventory Manual]. Beijing: The Chinese Medicine Electronic Audio and Video Publishing House. 2005.

[26] Bentler PM, Bonett DG. Significance tests and goodness of fit in the analysis of covariance structures. Psychol Bull. 1980,88:588 – 606.

[27] Hu LT, Bentler PM. Cutoff criteria for fit indexes in covariance structure analysis: conventional criteria versus new alternatives. Struct Equ Modeling. 1999,6:1 – 55.

[28] Fluss R, Faraggi D, Reiser B. Estimation of the Youden Index and its associated cutoff point. Biom J. 2005,47:458 – 472.

[29] Streiner DL. Starting at the beginning: an introduction to coefficient alpha and internal consistency. J Pers Assess. 2003,80:99 – 103.

[30] Karademas EC, Christopoulou S, Dimostheni A, Pavlu F. Health anxiety and cognitive interference: evidence from the application of a modified Stroop task in two studies. Pers Individ Dif. 2008,44:1138 – 1150.

[31] Boston AF, Merrick PL. Health anxiety among older people: an exploratory study of health anxiety and safety behaviors in a cohort of older adults in New Zealand. Int Psychogeriatr. 2010,22:549 – 558.

[32] Tang NK, Salkovskis PM, Poplavskaya E, Wright KJ, Hanna M, Hester J. Increased use of safety-seeking behaviors in chronic back pain patients with high health anxiety. Behav Res Ther. 2007,45:2821 – 2835.

[33] Seivewright H, Salkovskis P, Green J, et al. Prevalence and service implications of health anxiety in genitourinary medicine clinics. Int J STD AIDS. 2004,15:519 – 522.

[34] Kehler MD, Hadjistavropoulos HD. Is health anxiety a significant problem for individuals with multiple sclerosis? J Behav Med. 2009,32: 150 – 161.

[35] Rachman S. Health anxiety disorders: a cognitive construal. Behav Res Ther. 2012,50:502 – 512.

[36] Park SH, Goo JM, Jo CH. Receiver operating characteristic (ROC) curve: practical review for radiologists. Korean J Radiol. 2004,5:11 – 18.

[37] Tang NK, Wright KJ, Salkovskis PM. Prevalence and correlates of clinical insomnia co-occurring with chronic back pain. J Sleep Res. 2007, 16:85 – 95.

[38] Sulkowski ML, Mariaskin A, Storch EA. Obsessive-compulsive spectrum disorder symptoms in college students. J Am Coll Health. 2011,59: 342 – 348.

[39] Schreiber F, Neng JM, Heimlich C, Witthöft M, Weck F. Implicit affective evaluation bias in hypochondriasis: findings from the Affect Misattribution Procedure. J Anxiety Disord. 2014,28:671 – 678.

[40] Marcus DK, Hughes KT, Arnau RC. Health anxiety, rumination, and negative affect: a mediational analysis. J Psychosom Res. 2008,64: 495 – 501.

[41] Hart J, Björgvinsson T. Health anxiety and hypochondriasis: description and treatment issues highlighted through a case illustration. Bull Menninger Clin. 2010,74:122 – 140.

Supplementary materials:

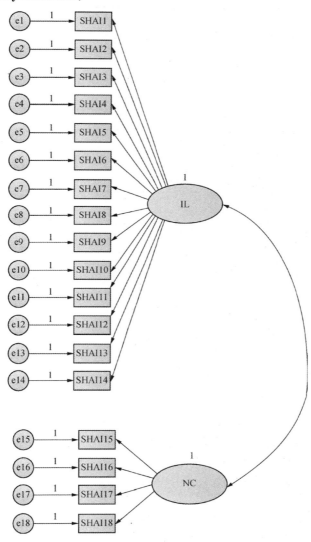

Figure S1   interrelationship between the two facets of health anxiety.

Notes: IL and NC are subscales of SHAI. SHAII to SHAII8 are object properties which represent each item; e1 to e18 are residual variables corresponding to each object properties.

Abbreviations: SHAI, Short Health Anxiety Inventory; IL, Illness Likelihood; NC, Negative Consequences.

Table S1 Correlations of Chinese-version SHAI Total With IL, NC, and each item

Item	SHAI	total	IL[a]	NC[a]
IL[a]	0.965**			
NC[a]	0.731**	0.526**		
1	0.590**	0.607**		
2	0.438**	0.460**		
3	0.417**	0.487**		
4	0.622**	0.638**		
5	0.700**	0.730**		
6	0.619**	0.640**		
7	0.597**	0.610**		
8	0.543**	0.570**		
9	0.564**	0.581**		
10	0.392**	0.417**		
11	0.679**	0.667**		
12	0.635**	0.664**		
13	0.462**	0.441**		
14	0.412**	0.428**		
15	0.564**			0.737**
16	0.504**			0.730**
17	0.545**			0.780**
18	0.505**			0.651**

Notes: [a]A subscale of SHAI. ** $P \leqslant 0.01$.

Abbreviations: SHAI, Short Health Anxiety Inventory; IL, Illness Likelihood; NC, Negative Consequences.

[作者及发表刊物:

Yuqun Zhang, Rui Liu, Guohong Li, Shengqin Mao, Yonggui Yuan. The reliability and validity of a Chinese-version short Health Anxiety Inventory: an investigation of university students[J]. Neuropschiatr Dis Treat. 2015,11:1739 - 1747.]

附:　　　　　　　　　**简式健康焦虑量表(SHAI)**

指导语:以下是一个问卷,由18道题组成,每一道题均有4句短句,代表4个可能的答案。请仔细阅读每一道题的所有回答(a～d)。读完后,从中选出一个最符合你情况的句子,在它后面对应的空格上打√。然后,再接着回答下一题。

题目	选项	
1.	(a) 我不担心我的健康	
	(b) 我偶尔担心我的健康	
	(c) 我花费很多时间担心我的健康	
	(d) 我花费绝大多数时间担心我的健康	
2.	(a) 相比大多数同龄人,我感受到的疼痛/痛苦少	
	(b) 相比大多数同龄人,我感受到的疼痛/痛苦相同	
	(c) 相比大多数同龄人,我感受到的疼痛/痛苦多	
	(d) 我总是感觉到疼痛/痛苦	
3.	(a) 我通常不会感受到身体的感觉或变化	
	(b) 我有时感受到身体的感觉或变化	
	(c) 我经常感受到身体的感觉或变化	
	(d) 我总是感受到身体的感觉或变化	
4.	(a) 对我来说,控制不想疾病的事从来不是个问题	
	(b) 对我来说,大多数时间可以控制不想疾病的事	
	(c) 我努力控制自己不想疾病的事,但时常不能奏效	
	(d) 我难以控制自己不想疾病的事以至于我放弃抵抗了	
5.	(a) 我通常不会担心自己患重病	
	(b) 我有时担心自己患重病	
	(c) 我经常担心自己患重病	
	(d) 我总是担心自己患重病	
6.	(a) 我脑海中不会浮现自己生病的画面	
	(b) 我脑海中有时浮现自己生病的画面	
	(c) 我脑海中经常浮现自己生病的画面	
	(d) 我脑海中一直呈现自己生病的画面	

题目	选项	
7.	(a) 对我来说,不想健康的事没有任何困难	
	(b) 对我来说,不想健康的事有时候会有困难	
	(c) 对我来说,不想健康的事经常会有困难	
	(d) 没有任何事物能让我不想健康的事	
8.	(a) 如果医生告诉我没有病,我就不再担心	
	(b) 如果医生告诉我没有病,开始我不担心,有时一段时间后又担心	
	(c) 如果医生告诉我没有病,开始我不担心,总是一段时间后又担心	
	(d) 如果医生告诉我没有病,我依然担心	
9.	(a) 如果听说某种疾病,我从不认为自己患这种病	
	(b) 如果听说某种疾病,我有时认为自己患这种病	
	(c) 如果听说某种疾病,我经常认为自己患这种病	
	(d) 如果听说某种疾病,我总是认为自己患这种病	
10.	(a) 如果身体有某种感觉或变化,我很少想它意味着什么	
	(b) 如果身体有某种感觉或变化,我经常想它意味着什么	
	(c) 如果身体有某种感觉或变化,我总是想它意味着什么	
	(d) 如果身体有某种感觉或变化,我必须弄清楚它意味着什么	
11.	(a) 我通常认为自己患重病的几率极小	
	(b) 我通常认为自己患重病的几率较小	
	(c) 我通常认为自己患重病的几率较大	
	(d) 我通常认为自己患重病的几率很大	
12.	(a) 我从不认为自己患重病	
	(b) 我有时认为自己患重病	
	(c) 我经常认为自己患重病	
	(d) 我总是认为自己患重病	
13.	(a) 如果发现一种不明原因的身体感觉,我可以想其他的事情	
	(b) 如果发现一种不明原因的身体感觉,我有时难以想其他的事情	
	(c) 如果发现一种不明原因的身体感觉,我经常难以想其他的事情	
	(d) 如果发现一种不明原因的身体感觉,我总是难以想其他的事情	

题目	选项	
14.	(a) 我的家人/朋友认为我不够关心自身健康	
	(b) 我的家人/朋友认为我能正常关心自身健康	
	(c) 我的家人/朋友认为我关心自身健康过度	
	(d) 我的家人/朋友认为我有疑病症	
15.	(a) 如果患重病,我仍然能很享受生活	
	(b) 如果患重病,我仍然能有些享受生活	
	(c) 如果患重病,我几乎不能享受生活	
	(d) 如果患重病,我完全不能享受生活	
16.	(a) 如果我患重病,现代医学很可能治愈我的病	
	(b) 如果我患重病,现代医学有可能治愈我的病	
	(c) 如果我患重病,现代医学不太可能治愈我的病	
	(d) 如果我患重病,现代医学不可能治愈我的病	
17.	(a) 重病会毁掉我生活的一些方面	
	(b) 重病会毁掉我生活的很多方面	
	(c) 重病会毁掉我生活的几乎所有方面	
	(d) 重病会毁掉我生活的一切	
18.	(a) 如果患重病,我不会觉得失去尊严	
	(b) 如果患重病,我觉得有失尊严	
	(c) 如果患重病,我觉得非常有失尊严	
	(d) 如果患重病,我觉得完全没有尊严	

多伦多述情障碍量表(TAS-20)的
信度和效度研究

摘　要

目的　评价 TAS-20 量表的信度和效度。

方法　使用 TAS-20 对 112 例正常人对照样本和 102 例精神病人样本进行评定。

结果　TAS-20 具有良好的心理测量特性,Cronbach α 系数在 0.581~0.739,TAS-20 各分量表的劈半相关系数在 0.558~0.803,TAS-20 各分最表得分在正常人对照样本和精神病人样本之间存在非常显著性差异。

结论　TAS-20 量表具有良好的信度和效度,值得推广使用。

关键词　信度;效度;激惹;抑郁;焦虑;大学生

述情障碍(alexitymia)自从 1972 年 Sifneos 命名以来,引起心身医学和精神病学研究者的广泛重视。1984 年 Taylor GJ 等制定了多伦多述情障碍量表(Toronto alexithymia scale-26, TAS-26)用于述情障碍的研究[1]。1991 年姚芳传等将 TAS-26 引入国内,并对大学生和医务人员进行评定,得到了国内较高文化人群的常模[2]。1994 年 Taylor GJ 等对 TAS-26 进行了修订,并公布了 TAS-20 版本(表5),经检验具有比 TAS-26 更高的信度和效度[3,4]。目前 TAS-20 已有数个国家的版本(如意大利、日本等),TAS-20 的中文版尚未见报道。作者将之引入国内,并对问卷的信度效度进行了研究。

1　对象和方法

1.1　对象

研究对象包括两组,一组是正常人对照样本,另一组是精神病人样本。正常人对照样本为 112 例,男 58 例,女 54 例;年龄 17~52 岁,平均年龄(26.8±

12.1)岁;大学生 52 例,医生 29 例,护士 12 例,工人 19 例。精神病人样本共 102 例,男 50 例,女 52 例,年龄 19～53 岁,平均年龄(32.6±13.4)岁;抑郁症 56 例,精神分裂症 29 例,神经症和心身疾病 17 例,所有患者均符合中国精神疾病分类方案与诊断标准第 2 版修订本(CCMD-2-R)中的诊断标准[5]。

1.2 方法

多伦多述情障碍量表(TAS-20)问卷经 Taylor GJ 同意,由本文第一作者翻译成中文,经两名精神科主任医师校阅后,对译文做了进一步校改。TAS-20 量表共 20 个条目,按 1～5 级评分,其中 4、5、10、18、19 等 12 个条目按反向评分。本量表包括三个因子:因子一(F1,难以识别自己的情感):1、3、6、7、9、13、14 共 7 条;因子二(F2,难以描述自己的情感):2、4、11、12、17 共 5 条;因子三(F3,外向性思维):5、8、10、15、16、18、19、20 共 8 条。

所有被试均采用个体测试,当场检查有无遗漏,以保证问卷有效。

2 结果

2.1 TAS-20 的信度分析

2.1.1 TAS-20 条目和各分量表总分的一致性分析

以被试的各分量表得分为效标,求出被试在各条目的得分与各分量表得分的 Pearson 相关,相关系数均在 0.246 以上(见表 1),说明条目与各分量表总分的一致性较好。

表 1 TAS-20 条目和各分量表总分的相关系数

F1	r_1	r_2	F2	r_1	r_2	F3	r_1	r_2
1	0.586**	0.669**	2	0.680**	0.662**	5	0.475**	0.459**
2	0.736**	0.704**	4	0.650**	0.531**	8	0.514**	0.427**
6	0.586**	0.698**	11	0.620**	0.626**	10	0.493**	0.422**
7	0.616**	0.770**	12	0.315**	0.603**	15	0.351**	0.436**
9	0.689**	0.691**	17	0.526**	0.670**	16	0.359**	0.470**
13	0.684**	0.727**				18	0.392**	0.393**
14	0.619**	0.685**				19	0.554**	0.414**
						20	0.446**	0.246**

注:r_1 为正常人对照样本,r_2 为精神病人样本;** $P_均$<0.05,** P<0.001。

2.1.2 同质性信度(Cronbach α 系数和劈半相关系数 r_s)(见表 2)。

表 2 同质性信度(Cronbach α 系数和劈半相关系数 r_s)

	F1		F2		F3	
	α	r_s	α	r_s	α	r_s
正常人对照样本	0.645	0.596	0.630	0.558	0.581	0.621
精神病人样本	0.739	0.637	0.694	0.701	0.679	0.803

2.1.3 重测信度

30 例大学生在首次完成 TAS-20 的 4 周后重测量了 TAS-20,重测相关系数(r)分别为:F1 为 0.782,F2 为 0.687,F3 为 0.893,$P_{均}$<0.01。

2.1.4 TAS-20 各分量表之间的相关性(见表 3)。

表 3 TAS-20 各分量表之间的相关性

	F1	F2	F3
F1		0.715**	0.337**
F2	0.416**		0.422**
F3	0.695**	0.612**	

注:上面是精神病人样本组,** P<0.001。

2.2 TAS-20 问卷的区分效度

不同群体 TAS-20 各分量表得分情况比较(见表 4)。

表 4 不同群体 TAS-20 各分量表得分情况比较

	正常人对照样本组	精神病人样本组	t	P
F1	13.92±0.35	12.15±2.63	4.272	0.000
F2	21.68±3.40	20.49±3.68	2.440	0.015
F3	54.03±9.96	48.45±7.70	4.554	0.000

表5 多伦多述情障碍量表(TAS‑20)

请标明下面20个陈述句在何种程度符合您的情况。您可在"1. 很不同意;2. 不同意;3. 部分同意,部分不同意;4. 同意;5. 很同意"之中选择一项,请在相应的数字上画圈。

	很不同意	不同意	部分同意	同意	很同意
1. 我常常搞不清自己有什么样的感受。	1	2	3	4	5
2. 我感到难以用恰当的词语来描述我的感受。	1	2	3	4	5
3. 我有一些即使是医生也不能理解的身体感觉。	1	2	3	4	5
*4. 我能容易地描述出自己的感受。	1	2	3	4	5
*5. 我更喜欢分析问题而不仅仅是描述它们。	1	2	3	4	5
6. 当我心里难受时,我不知道究竟是悲伤、害怕、还是恼怒。	1	2	3	4	5
7. 我常常被我身体的一些感觉所困惑。	1	2	3	4	5
8. 我偏向于任事情发生,而不是去了解它们为何会发展成那样。	1	2	3	4	5
9. 我有一些自己难以识别的感受。	1	2	3	4	5
*10. 知道自己有何内心体验对我来说很重要。	1	2	3	4	5
11. 我难以描述我对别人有何感受。	1	2	3	4	5
12. 人们要我多描述一些我的感受。	1	2	3	4	5
13. 我不知道自己内心在发生一些什么活动。	1	2	3	4	5
14. 我常常不知道我为何会气愤。	1	2	3	4	5
15. 我喜欢与别人谈论他们的日常活动而不是他们的感受。	1	2	3	4	5
16. 我喜欢看"轻松"的娱乐片胜过看关于个人命运的情节片。	1	2	3	4	5
17. 即使是对密友,我也难以表露我内心深处的感受。	1	2	3	4	5
*18. 我能感到与某人有亲切感,即使在我们沉默无言之时。	1	2	3	4	5
*19. 我觉得省察自己的感受对于解决个人问题是有用的。	1	2	3	4	5
20. 寻找电影或戏剧中隐藏的意义会使人从娱乐中分心。	1	2	3	4	5

注:*条为反向评分。

3 讨论

述情障碍(alexitymia)又译作"情感表达不能"或"情感难言症",它并非一种独立的精神疾病,可为一种人格特征,也可为某些躯体或精神疾病时较常见到的心理特点,或为其继发症状[1]。述情障碍的检测和评定是很困难的。随着对述情障碍研究的增多,国外逐渐发展起来不少评定述情障碍的量表,如 Beth Israel 医院心身问卷(Sifneos 等,1972),Schalling Sifneos 人格量表(1979),MMPI 述情障碍量表(Kleiger,1980)、多伦多述情障碍量表(TAS‐26)(Taylor,1984)等[6]。但在 TAS‐26 的使用过程中,量表的缺点渐渐显露出来了。比如两个因子具有高度相关性,并且有几个条目在两个因子中具有显著的跨因子负荷;缺乏幻想因子的组成条目与全部 TAS 的条目总的相关系数较低,并且这个因子与 F1 呈负相关。另有研究发现,缺乏幻想因子与评因子与 F1 呈负相关。另有研究发现,缺乏幻想因子与评估情感意识和外向性思维的因子存在负相关,提示评估缺乏幻想的条目与述情障碍的其他因子间缺乏理论上的一致性[3]。故 Tayler 等对 TAS‐26 进行了修订,并于1994年公布了 TAS‐20 版本,经检验具有很好的信度和效度,并且避免了 TAS‐26 的缺陷。它由三个因子组成,F1 缺乏识别情感的能力,F2 缺乏描绘情感的能力,F3 外向性思维[3,4]。

TAS‐20 中文版的信度研究结果显示,TAS‐20 各分量表的重测相关系数为 0.687～0.893,表明该量表具有很好的跨时间稳定性。IDA 各分量表的条目与各分量表总分相关系数均在 0.246～0.770,同质性信度 Cronbach α 系数在 0.581～0.739,表明条目与各分量测试内容一致性较好。另外,IDA 各分量表的劈半相关系数在 0.558～0.803,也达到了心理计量学要求。

在效度方面,TAS‐20 分量表得分在正常人对照样本和精神病人样本患者 IDA 各分量表之间存在非常显著性差异,这说明 TAS‐20 量表的区分效度也达到了要求。

参考文献

[1] 姚芳传.述情障碍.国外医学精神病学分册,1991,18(3):141-144.

[2] 姚芳传,徐长宽,陈启豹,等.多伦多述情障碍量表对大学生和医务人员的评定.中国心理卫生杂志,1992,6(5):217-218.

[3] Bagby RM, Parker JDA, Taylor GJ. The tweny-item Toronto alexithymia scale-Ⅰ. Item selection and cross-validaion of the factor structuire. J Paychosom Res, 1994,38 (1):23-32.

[4] Bagby RM, Taylor GJ, Parker JDA. The tweny-item Toronto alexithymia scale-Ⅱ. Convergent, discriminant, and concurrent validiy. J Psychosom Res,1994,38, 33-40. Taylor GJ. Recent developments in alexithymia theory and research. Can J Paychiatry, 2000,45 (1):134-142

[5] 中华医学会精神科学会,南京医科大学脑科医院.中国精神疾病分类方案与诊断标准第2版修订本(CCMD-2-R).南京:东南大学出版社,1995.

[6] YUAN YC. Current Status of Alexithymia in China. Chin J Clin Rehabilitation, 2002, 6(18):2822-2824.

[作者及发表刊物:

袁勇贵,沈鑫华,张向荣,吴爱勤,孙厚纯,张宁,张心保,李海林.多伦多述情障碍量表(TAS-20)的信度和效度研究[J].四川精神卫生,2013,16(1):25-27.]

激惹、抑郁和焦虑量表(IDA)的
信度和效度研究

摘 要

目的：评价 IDA 量表的信度和效度。

方法：使用 IDA、SDS 和 SAS 对 291 例大学生和 64 例抑郁症患者进行评定。

结果：IDA 具有良好的心理测量特性，Cronbach α 系数在 0.419—0.769，IDA 各分量表的劈半相关系数在 0.427—0.639，IDA 各分量表与 SDS、SAS 间的相关系数均在 0.400—0.776，IDA 各分量表得分在非抑郁大学生、抑郁大学生和抑郁症患者之间存在非常显著性差异。

结论：IDA 量表具有良好的信度和效度，值得推广使用。

关键词：信度；效度；激惹；抑郁；焦虑；大学生

激惹、抑郁和焦虑量表(irritability, depression and anxiety scale, IDA)是 Saith RP 于 1978 年提出的[1]。这是首次试图在抑郁/焦虑患者中区分出易激惹症状因子的量表设计(见附表)，它包括 18 个项目的 4 级量表，其中 5 项评定抑郁，5 项评定焦虑，另外为激惹性增设的外显表现和内心体验各 4 项。鉴于国内尚无评定激惹症状的量表，故作者将之引入国内，并对问卷的信度效度进行了研究。

1 对象与方法

1.1 对象

研究对象包括两组，一组是大学生被试，另一组是抑郁症患者。大学生组为某医科大学本科一年级学生 291 例，其中男 196 例，女 95 例，年龄 17～

22岁,平均年龄(19.8±2.1)岁。抑郁症组共64例,其中男29例,女35例,年龄19~67岁,平均年龄(42.9±13.4)岁,均符合中国精神疾病分类方案与诊断标准第2版修订本(CCMD-2-R)中抑郁症的诊断标准[2]。

1.2 方法

1.2.1 激惹、抑郁和焦虑量表(IDA)

IDA问卷经Saith RP同意,由本文第一作者翻译成中文,经两名精神科主任医师校阅后,对译文做了进一步校改。IDA量表共18个条目,每个条目相当于一个有关症状;按0—3级评分,其中3,4,6,7,8,9,10,11,14,15,16,18等12个条目按反向评分。本量表包括四个因子:因子一(抑郁)包括1,3,5,9,12等五个条目;因子二(焦虑)包括2,7,10,14,17等五个条目;因子三(内向性激惹)包括8,11,15,18等四个条目;因子四(外向性激惹)包括4,6,13,16等四个条目。

1.2.2 抑郁自评量表(SDS)[3]

由Zung于1965年编制的,为自评量表,由20个陈述句组成,每一条目相当于一个有关症状;按1~4级评分。

1.2.3 焦虑自评量表(SAS)[3]

由Zung于1971年编制的,为自评量表,由20个陈述句组成,每一条目相当于一个有关症状;按1~4级评分。

对大学生被试采用集体问卷调查,当场回收;对抑郁症患者采取个体测试。

2 结果

2.1 IDA的信度分析

2.1.1 IDA条目和各分量表总分的一致性分析

以被试的各分量表得分为效标,求出被试在各条目的得分与各分量表得分的Pearson相关,相关系数均在0.360以上(表1),说明条目与各分量表总分的一致性较好。

表 1　IDA 条目和各分量表总分的相关系数

D 条目	r_1	r_2	A 条目	r_1	r_2	I 条目	r_1	r_2	O 条目	r_1	r_2
1	0.622	0.810	2	0.469	0.593	8	0.734	0.822	4	0.686	0.607
3	0.551	0.652	7	0.592	0.663	11	0.726	0.770	6	0.705	0.771
5	0.606	0.714	10	0.500	0.738	15	0.479	0.545	13	0.427	0.718
9	0.564	0.587	14	0.551	0.678	18	0.606	0.698	16	0.596	0.666
12	0.528	0.711	17	0.572	0.360						

注:r_1 为大学生样本,r_2 为抑郁症样本;$P_均$<0.001.

2.1.2　同质性信度(Cronbach α 系数和劈半相关系数 r_s)(见表2)。

表 2　同质性信度(Cronbach α 系数和劈半相关系数 r_s)

	D		A		I		O	
	α	r_s	α	r_s	α	r_s	α	r_s
学生组	0.545	0.516	0.419	0.456	0.591	0.496	0.535	0.529
患者组	0.769	0.639	0.541	0.427	0.704	0.621	0.665	0.581

2.1.3　重测信度

31 例大学生在首次完成 IDA 的 4 周后重测量了 IDA,重测相关系数(r)分别为:D 为 0.488,A 为 0.524,I 为 0.493,O 为 0.761,$P_均$<0.05。

2.1.4　IDA 各分量表之间的相关性(见表3)。

表 3　IDA 各分量表之间的相关性

	学生组			患者组		
	D	A	I	D	A	I
A	0.375			0.646		
I	0.365	0.487		0.424	0.476	
O	0.310	0.347	0.450	0.452	0.524	0.498

注:$P_均$<0.001。

2.2 IDA 问卷的效度分析

2.2.1 IDA 的聚合效度（见表 4）。

表 4 学生组和患者组 IDA 各分量表与 SDS、SAS 间的相关性

		D	A	I	O
学生组	SDS	0.564	0.462	0.557	0.405
	SAS	0.507	0.442	0.481	00400
患者组	SDS	0.776	0.655	0.556	0.474
	SAS	0.693	0.716	0.502	0.541

注：$P_{均}$<0.001。

2.2.2 区分效度

按 SDS 评分≥50 将大学生分成两组，即抑郁学生组和非抑郁学生组。不同群体 IDA 各分量表得分情况比较（见表 5）。

表 5 不同群体 IDA 各分量表得分情况比较

	非抑郁学生组(n=241)	抑郁学生组(n=50)	患者组(n=64)
D	3.08±1.57	5.24±2.27**	8.78±3.56**##
A	4.63±2.11	6.48±1.95**	8.45±2.96**##
I	2.83±1.72	5.30±2.64**	5.09±2.88**
O	2.63±1.63	4.10±2.46**	4.23±2.80**

注：** 与非抑郁学生比较，P<0.001；## 与抑郁学生比较，P<0.001。

3 讨论

激惹(irritability)是焦虑的核心成分之一，但激惹作为一种与焦虑和其他情感(如抑郁)有关的重要症状在临床工作中常常被忽略了[4]。Snaith 等在 1978 年首次使用 IDA 量表对激惹进行评估，发现 IDA 量表具有很好的信度和效度[1]。

信度研究结果显示，IDA 各分量表的重测相关系数为 0.488～0.761，表明该量表具有很好的跨时间稳定性。IDA 各分量表的条目与各分量表总分

相关系数均在 0.360～0.810,同质性信度 Cronbach α 系数在 0.419～0.769,表明条目与各分量表测试内容一致性较好。另外,IDA 各分量表的劈半相关系数在 0.427～0.639,也达到了心理计量学要求。

在效度方面,不论是大学生还是抑郁症患者,IDA 各分量表与 SDS、SAS 间的相关系数均在 0.400～0.776,说明 IDA 各分量表的聚合效度较好。IDA 各分量表得分在非抑郁大学生、抑郁大学生和抑郁症患者之间存在非常显著性差异,D 和 A 分量表对抑郁大学生和抑郁症患者也能进行比较好的区分,后者得分显著高于前者,这说明 IDA 量表的区分效度也达到了要求。

参考文献

[1] Snaith RP, Taylor CM. Irritability: definition, assessment and associated factors. Br J Psychiatr,1985,147(2):127-136.

[2] 中华医学会精神科学会,南京医科大学脑科医院.中国精神疾病分类方案与诊断标准第 2 版修订本(CCMD-2-R).南京:东南大学出版社,1995:69-70.

[3] 张明园.精神科评定量表手册.长沙:湖南科学技术出版社,1993:34-41.

[4] Tyrer P. Anxiey: a multidisciplinay review. London: Imperial College Press, 1999:24-34.

[作者及发表刊物:

袁勇贵,沈鑫华,吴爱勤,孙厚纯,张心保,李海林.激惹、抑郁和焦虑量表(IDA)的信度和效度研究[J].四川精神卫生,2002,15(1):11-13.]

附： <center>**激惹、抑郁、焦虑自评量表**</center>

指导语:本量表的目的是评估您最近1周的感觉,请按顺序阅读每一道题,在最适合您的答案下打勾。每题只选一个答案,请回答全部问题。

1. 我感到高兴

□我很高兴　　□有时高兴　　□很少高兴　　□一点也不高兴

2. 我能坐下来,并且感到很轻松

□完全能做到　　　　　□有时能做到

□不能完全做到　　　　□一点也做不到

*3. 我的胃口

□非常差　　□较差　　□很好　　□非常好

*4. 我经常发脾气,并且怒斥别人

□经常是　　□有时是　　□不完全这样　　□从不这样

5. 我能笑,并且很开心

□是这样的　　□有时是这样　　□很少这样　　□从未这样

*6. 我感到我可能会失去控制,并且会伤害别人

□有时　　□偶尔　　□很少　　□从来不

*7. 我胃部不适

□经常这样　　□有时这样　　□很少这样　　□从未有过

*8. 我脑中有自伤的想法

□有时有　　□很少有　　□几乎没有　　□从未有过

*9. 我早醒

□2个小时以上　　　　□大约1小时

□少于1小时　　　　　□睡眠正常

*10. 我感觉到紧张

□经常紧张　　□有时紧张　　□很少紧张　　□从不紧张

*11. 我可能会伤害自己的感情

　　□肯定会　　　□有时会　　　□很少会　　　□绝不会

12. 我保持原有兴趣

　　□绝大部分仍存在　　　　□部分存在

　　□很少存在　　　　　　　□完全不存在

13. 我有耐心与别人相处

　　□全部时间　　　　　　　□绝大部分时间

　　□部分时间　　　　　　　□从没有过耐心与人相处

*14. 无缘无故地恐慌或惊恐

　　□经常有　　□有时有　　　□很少有　　　□从没有过

*15. 我对自己或听到我的名字就恼火

　　□经常是这样　　　　　　□有时是这样

　　□不常这样　　　　　　　□从没有过

*16. 人们使我心烦意乱,以致于我要损门或摔东西

　　□经常是　　□有时　　　□偶尔　　　□从来没有

17. 我独自外出,不感到紧张

　　□是的　　　□有时是　　□很少　　　□从没有过

*18. 最近,我对自己感到不满

　　□一直这样　□经常这样　□很少这样　□从未这样

注:* 为反向评分。

袁勇贵主任已出版的著作

1. 2006 年　袁勇贵　唐勇·主编　《精神科门急诊手册》
   （江苏科学技术出版社）

2. 2006 年　袁勇贵·主编　《远离灰色——谈抑郁情绪管理》
   （东南大学出版社）

3. 2007 年　袁勇贵　郑爱民　陶领纲·主编
   《远离失眠——谈睡眠障碍管理》（东南大学出版社）

4. 2008 年　袁勇贵　杨忠·主编
   《远离焦虑——谈焦虑情绪管理》（东南大学出版社）

5. 2008 年　袁勇贵　杨忠　曹音·主编
   《远离痴呆——谈记忆障碍管理》（东南大学出版社）

6. 2008 年　袁勇贵·主编　《精神医学案例习题集》
   （东南大学出版社）

7. 2008 年　吴爱勤　袁勇贵　袁国桢　·主编
   《医疗机构医务人员"三基"训练指南(精神科)》
   （东南大学出版社）

8. 2009 年　吴爱勤　袁勇贵　袁国桢·主编
   《医疗机构医务人员"三基"训练习题集(精神科)》
   （东南大学出版社）

9. 2013 年　袁勇贵·主编　《快速识别心理障碍》

（东南大学出版社）

10. 2014 年　方建群　袁勇贵·主编
《人格心理学学习指导及习题集》（人民卫生出版社）

11. 2014 年　袁勇贵·主编　《抑郁障碍共病:理论与实践》

（东南大学出版社）

12. 2015 年　袁勇贵　徐治·主编　《自我识别心理障碍》

（东南大学出版社）

13. 2015 年　吴爱勤　袁勇贵·主编
《中国当代心身医学研究(1994～2014)》

（东南大学出版社）

14. 2016 年　袁勇贵　李英辉·主编　《健康心理与长寿人生》

（中国协和医科大学出版社）

15. 2016 年　袁勇贵·主编　《中国卒中后抑郁障碍规范化诊疗指南》

（东南大学出版社）

16. 2018 年　袁勇贵·等著　《平衡心理治疗》（东南大学出版社）

17. 2018 年　袁勇贵·等著　《袁·说》（东南大学出版社）

18. 2018 年　袁勇贵·等著　《心身医学新理念》（东南大学出版社）